Endoscopy in Neuro-Otology

# Endoscopy in Neuro-Otology

**Jacques Magnan, M. D.**
Professor of Otolaryngology
Hôpıtaux de Marseille
Marseille, France

**Mario Sanna, M. D.**
Professor of Otolaryngology
University of Chieti
Chieti, Italy
Instituto Scientifico Ospedale San Rafaelle
Rome, Italy
Gruppo Otologico
Piacenza, Italy

With the collaboration of

**Jean-Pierre Bebear, M. D.**
Centre Hospitalier
Universitaire de Bordeaux
Bordeaux, France

**André Chays, M. D.**
Hôpital Nord
Marseille, France

**Nadine Girard, M. D.**
Hôpital Nord
Marseille, France

**G. O'Donoghue, M. D.**
Queen's Medical Centre
University Hospital
Nottingham, England

**Charles Raybaud, M. D.**
Hôpital Nord
Marseille, France

and

L. Broder, M. Bruzzo, F. Caces, V. Darrouzet, Hani El Garem, Alessandra Russo, Abdel Taibah

345 illustrations

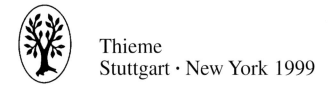

Thieme
Stuttgart · New York 1999

*Library of Congress Cataloging-in-Publication Data*
Magnan, Jacques.
Endoscopy in neuro-otology/ Jacques Magnan, Mario Sanna
with the collaboration of Jean-Pierre Bebear...[et al .].
     p. cm.
Includes bibliographical references and index.
ISBN 3-13-113061 - X (GTV). — ISBN 0-86577-828-0 (TNY)
1. Cerebellopontile angle—Endoscopic surgery. 2. Ear—
Endoscopic surgery. 3. Endoscopic surgery. 4. Otology. I. Sanna,
M. II. Title.
     [DNLM: 1. Cerebellopontine Angle—surgery. 2. Surgical
Procedures, Endoscopic. 3. Otologic Surgical Procedures.
WL 320 M 196e 1999 ]
RF 126. M34 1999
617.8'059—dc21
DNLM/DLC
for Library of Congress                                            98-32395
                                                                          Cip

*Important Note:* Medicine is an ever-changing science undergoing continual development. Research and clinical experience are continually expanding our knowledge, in particular our knowledge of proper treatment and drug therapy. Insofar as this book mentions any dosage or application, readers may rest assured that the authors, editors, and publishers have made every effort to ensure that such references are in accordance with the state of knowledge at the time of production of the book.

Nevertheless this does not involve, imply, or express any guarantee or responsibility on the part of the publishers in respect of any dosage instructions and forms of application stated in the book. Every user is requested to examine carefully the manufacturers' leaflets accompanying each drug and to check, if necessary in consultation with a physician or specialist, whether the dosage schedules mentioned therein or the contraindications stated by the manufacturers differ from the statements made in the present book. Such examination is particularly important with drugs that are either rarely used or have been newly released on the market. Every dosage schedule or every form of application used is entirely at the user's own risk and responsibility. The authors and publishers request every user to report to the publishers any discrepancies or inaccuracies noticed.

*Additional Collaborators*

L. Broder, M. D.
Hôpitaux de Marseille
Marseille, France

Hani El Garem, M. D.
Hôpital Nord
Marseille, France

M. Bruzzo, M. D.
Hôpitaux de Marseille
Marseille, France

Alessandra Russo, M.D.
Gruppo Otologico
Piacenza, Italy

F. Caces, M. D.
Hôpitaux de Marseille
Marseille, France

Abdel Taibah, M.D.
Gruppo Otologico
Piacenza, Italy

V. Darrouzet, M. D.
Universitaire de Bordeaux
Bordeaux, France

© 1999 Georg Thieme Verlag, Rüdigerstraße 14,
D-70469 Stuttgart, Germany
Thieme New York, 333 Seventh Avenue,
New York, NY 10001 USA.

Typesetting and Photolitho: Before S.r.l.,
Grottammare (AP), Italy

Printed in Germany by Staudigl Druck, Donauwörth

Cover design by Renate Stockinger, Stuttgart

ISBN 3-13-113061-X (GTV)
ISBN 0-86577-828-O (TNY)                              1 2 3 4 5 6

# Foreword

The authors have to be commended for writing this brilliant overview on the application of endoscopy in the field of neuro-otology.

It is not by chance that Professor J. Magnan is one of the initiators of this book. In the early '70s I visited Marseille to assist with a vestibular neurectomy performed through a minimal retrosigmoid keyhole approach by Magnan's teacher, Professor G. Bremond. The apple does not fall far from the tree: the enthusiasm for keyhole endoscopic surgery originated at that time in Marseille.

The first chapter of this volume on endoscopic technology is extremely accurate and practical. The second chapter on endoscopic anatomy of the cerebellopontine angle is fascinating because it shows how the endoscope unveils details of neural and vascular anatomy that escape microscopic exploration. One senses immediately the enthusiasm felt by the authors in discovering a new endoscopic world and the effort made to describe this with scientific precision.

The last chapter deals with the application of endoscopic techniques in neuro-otologic surgery. The authors show a very balanced judgement in their indications and present a concise review of the advantages of endoscopy as the main technique, or as an adjuvant to the microscope, in solving difficult surgical problems. The illustrations used to demonstrate the various procedures are most impressive. I am sure that this superb volume will have a lasting impact on the future development of neuro-otology and skull base surgery.

*Ugo Fisch, M.D.*
Director
Clinic for Ear, Nose, and Throat Surgery
University Hospital Zürich

# Contents

# 1 Endoscope Technology

## Introduction

Endoscopy is now firmly established as a major investigative and therapeutic technology in a wide range of disciplines. The speciality of otolaryngology and head and neck surgery owes its existence to the particular difficulties encountered when examining the dark recesses of the head and neck. It is therefore not surprising that the speciality has been at the forefront of developments in endoscopic techniques for use in this anatomical area. In the field of otolaryngology, rhinologists were quick to welcome the endoscope for use in the management of sinus disorders; by contrast, otologists and skull base surgeons have been less than enthusiastic, despite the wide range of possible applications in this area.

This book presents ways in which endoscopic technology can be applied in the new field of neuro-otology and skull base surgery.

## History of Endoscopy in the Cerebellopontine Angle

The first comprehensive description of endoscopy in the cerebellopontine angle (CPA) was provided by the French surgeon Doyen (1917), who described an endoscopic technique for selective fifth nerve section in trigeminal neuralgia. His description is worth quoting: "The occipital bone was perforated with a 20 mm burr, the dura was opened and the cerebellum retracted; an intracranial endoscope was then introduced, showing the trigeminal root about 5–6 mm above the acusticus and about 14 or 15 mm beyond it." He described a speculum specially developed for this purpose, which he inserted between the posterior surface of the petrous bone and the cerebellum, as well as a special guillotine neurotomy knife designed to protect the motor fibers of the trigeminal nerve during neurotomy. Another description of this technique was given by Prott (1974), advocating a transmastoid retrolabyrinthine approach to the CPA. Oppel and Mulch (1979) described a similar approach for selective trigeminal root section. However, the range of instruments available until relatively recently was a major deterrent to progress, and the approach attracted few researchers.

The endoscopic anatomy of the CPA has been described by O'Donoghue and O'Flynn (1993). Using a range of sinus endoscopes (0°, 25°, and 110°), they examined the CPA in ten fresh cadavers. They described four anatomical levels:

Level 1. The uppermost level, which holds the trigeminal and abducent nerves and their related vascular structures (usually the superior cerebellar artery and vein).
Level 2. This contains the neurovascular acousticofacial bundle, and is situated approximately 55 mm deep to the retrosigmoid craniotomy site (the loops of the anterior inferior cerebellar artery were clearly visualized, and their relationship to the neural structures and the porus acusticus was extremely variable).
Level 3. This contains the ninth, tenth, and eleventh cranial nerves and related vascular structures (usually the posterior inferior cerebellar artery).
Level 4. This is at the level of the foramen magnum; it contains the spinal root of the accessory and hypoglossal nerves, and the vertebral, basilar, and posterior inferior cerebellar arteries.

O'Donoghue and O'Flynn emphasized the importance of obtaining experience and training with cadaver models before endoscopes are used in the operating room.

McKennan (1993) described the use of an endoscope for viewing the lateral recesses of the internal auditory canal to verify complete excision of an acoustic tumor and continuity of the facial and cochlear nerves. The use of angled rigid endoscopes in neuroendoscopy improved the degree of surgical exposure possible in this difficult-to-reach area.

Papers by Magnan et al. (1993, 1994) stimulated renewed interest in endoscopic surgery in the CPA with the use of contemporary endoscopes and videoendoscopic equipment. The authors used a rigid instrument with 0° viewing, a diameter of 4 mm, and a length of 6 cm. They found that a major advantage of the endoscope was that, with its wide angle of illumination, it was able to provide a complete panoramic view of the neurovascular relationships in the angle, without the need for retraction or dissection. To maintain the sterility of the endoscope, an immersible sterilizable video camera was attached to it, and the advancement of the instrument can thus be checked on a video monitor.

The fundamental importance of the endoscopic procedure is that it allows a more comprehensive map of the neurovascular components to be obtained without the need for cerebellar retraction. Incorporating the endoscope into the standard surgical armamentarium in the field of neuro-otology has made an important contribution to the minimally invasive surgery approach–offering patients the potential for minimal morbidity.

# Endoscopic Equipment

Major advances in the development of endoscopic devices (in addition to the electric light bulb and telescope optics) were made in the 1950s and 1960s with the invention of Hopkins rod lens optical design for rigid endoscopes; fiber-optic light cables; cold light sources; imaging fiber optics for flexible endoscopes; video for viewing and documentation; and surgical instruments for therapeutic endoscopic procedures.

## Optical Imaging System

The word "endoscopy" is derived from Greek, and basically means "looking into." The development of the endoscope met a long-felt need in medicine to be able to observe organs within the body, either through the natural bodily openings or small artificially made openings. The development of "keyhole" approaches in surgery allowed a move from more invasive to less invasive methods of treatment.

Decisive improvements in the image quality provided by rigid endoscopes were achieved by the English physicist H.H. Hopkins in the mid-1960s, with the development and application of so called "rod" lenses. Rod lenses differed from the existing achromatic lenses in that their length is several times greater than their diameter. Named after Hopkins, the rod lens design was adopted and further developed in the manufacture of endoscopes, allowing optimization of optical transmission across a wide range of parameters (depth of field, absence of distortion, brightness of the image) (O'Donoghue et al. 1994).

The relationship between the diameter and the length of an endoscope requires a complex optical imaging system (Figs. **1–3**). The intermediate image produced by the lens is transported through a series of rod lens inversion systems over the length of the endoscope sheath. The term "inversion system" indicates that each one of these systems inverts the image. The image is always returned to the correct position if there is an even number of rod lenses in the system.

The intermediate image from the last proximal inversion system is shown enlarged through the eyepiece. Hopkins telescopes are distinguished by their great depth of field, with simultaneous high resolution and contrast reproduction, and they have set the standard for all rigid endoscopic imaging for many years. The standardized eyepiece on the proximal side of the endoscope allows specialized video cameras to be connected, so that images can be recorded and displayed on a monitor.

The variable direction of view is of practical importance for rigid endoscopes. The direction of view describes the angle between the symmetrical axis of the telescope and the middle axis of the view. In neuro-otology, the safest endoscope is 6 cm long, 4 mm in diameter, and has an angle of 0° (Karl Storz GmbH, Hopkins Telescope 1215 AA). This provides a panoramic view directed towards the front, which

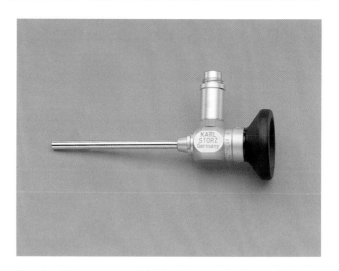

Fig. **1**   Tele-otoscope with Hopkins straight forward-viewing lens, 0°, diameter 4 mm, length 6 cm.

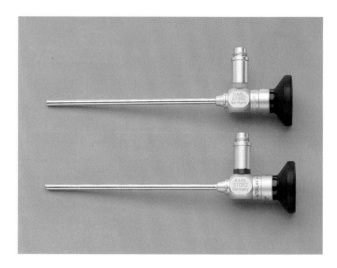

Fig. **2**   *Above*: straight forward-viewing telescope, 0°, diameter 4 mm, length 11 cm. *Below*: forward-oblique telescope, 30°, diameter 4 mm, length 11 cm.

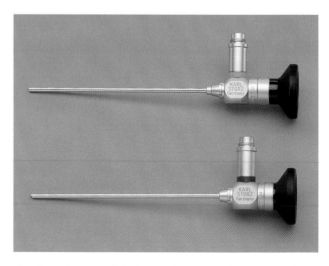

Fig. **3**   *Above*: straight forward-viewing telescope, 0°, diameter 2.7 mm, length 11 cm. *Below*: forward-oblique telescope, 30°, diameter 2.7 mm.

remains unchanged during the rotation of the telescope. The limited length prevents inadvertent contact with deeper structures.

Other useful endoscopes are 11 cm long and 4 mm and 2.7 mm in diameter, with an angle of 30°. Rotating the 30° telescope around the longitudinal axis changes the field of vision, in contrast to 0° one, and allows the surgeon to look around corners (Karl Storz GmbH, Hopkins Telescope 1216 BA and 7208 BA).

The 70° and 120° endoscopes allow lateral viewing, but are dangerous in the cerebellopontine angle, since the surgeon cannot appreciate the exact position of the endoscope tip. We therefore do not recommend them.

## Light Sources (Fig. 4)

Endoscopic illumination is provided by three separate devices: a remote light source, a flexible fiber-optic light cable that connects the light source to the telescope, and the fiber-optics within the endoscope, which transmit the illumination light from the endoscope tip to the image plane.

Three types of light sources, or lamps, are in regular use in endoscopy today: tungsten halogen, metal halide, and xenon short arc. Karl Storz have designed devices using each of these three lamps. The choice is determined by the cost and size of the instrument, and, most importantly, by the brightness and whiteness of the light required for viewing and documenting the procedure.

## Video for Viewing and Recording

Video cameras are lightweight cubes 2–3 cm in size, which produce computer-enhanced images of high resolution and contrast in vivid true color. Video images are routinely shown on multiple monitors in the operating room, so that the whole surgical team can participate in the procedure. Documentation is easily carried out using video recorders and the new single-image electronic processors, which allow single images to be digitally stored and printed out later.

Several types of video cameras are available (Figs. 5, 6). Three-chips cameras have individual chips for each of the primary colors, producing extremely high resolution images with excellent color fidelity. The digital electronics contained in the camera controller have automatic exposure and color control; automatic white balance; digital contrast enhancement; zoom lenses from 20 to 50 mm; and a built-in character generator. This type of camera has keys on its head allowing control of camera functions and the video recorder/printer. The camera can be mounted on all telescope eyepieces, and can be adapted to operating microscopes. The entire camera head can be gas-sterilized or soaked in high-level disinfectant. It has a world power supply, and is available in both PAL and NTSC formats.

Single-chip cameras are also available at lower cost, and these are very satisfactory for operating

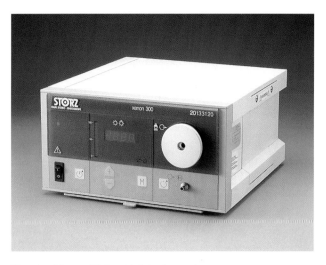

Fig. 4 Xenon 300 cold light fountain.

room use. Many of the optical and electronic features are the same as those in the three-chips cameras. Both camera-systems are available with Integrated Processing Module (IPM) including the functions of the Digivideo.

There are also additional electronic devices which enhance the performance of Karl Storz video cameras. The Digivideo is a system that digitizes the entire image and processes it for contrast enhancement in real time. This process significantly improves the ability to recognize details in the image. The Twinvideo system provides two simultaneous images on the monitor–either from two cameras, attached to endoscopes or mounted on the operating microscope; or a video image and a radiographic or ultrasound image; or a real-time video and a recorded image from a previous procedure.

In most modern operating rooms, the entire endoscopic video system is assembled on a cart in order to eliminate the clutter of electrical cords and interconnecting cables. Carts with lockable wheels are available for fixed mounting of the monitors, or the monitors can be mounted on adjustable arms. Shelves pro-

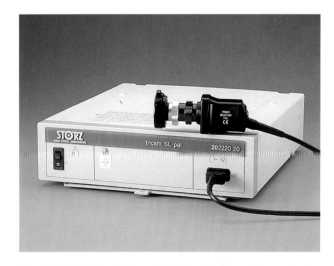

Fig. 5 Endovision Tricam SL-IPM, with three-chips technology color system (PAL/ NTSC).

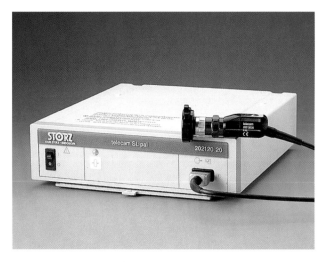

Fig. **6**    Endovision Telecam SL-IPM with Integrated Image Processing Module, that includes the Digivideo.

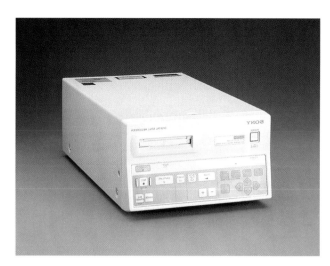

Fig. **7**    Digital Still Recorder for direct image capture from a video camera.

vide room for the light source, video camera controller, and recorder, Digivideo and Twinvideo, Digital Still Recorder (Fig. **7**), and printer, adaptors for attaching the video camera to an operating microscope, a still film camera, and a photo-flash module for special documentation. All components of the video system are permanently interconnected on the cart, and the entire system can be readily moved from one operating room to another.

## Sterilization of Endoscopic Equipment

Endoscopic instruments require gentle handling and special care during cleaning, disinfection, and sterilization processes.

Telescopes should be cleaned immediately after use. To avoid damage, they should be immersed individually, and the telescope should be held by firmly grasping the eyepiece end; they should never be handled using the distal end alone. The stainless-steel sheath should never be bent, as this could lead to breakage or cracks in the rod lens system. The telescope should be handled with care. Hard knocks, particularly at the distal end, may result in damage to the telescope or cracking and allow liquid, steam, and other materials to penetrate it. If this happens, the damage will cause a foggy or blurred image area.

Light cable adaptors should be removed prior to cleaning. The lens and the fiber-optic inlet set must be cleaned with alcohol wipes or sterile cotton-tipped applicators, using 70% alcohol.

Water of at least drinking quality must be used to rinse the telescope. Compressed air or a soft cloth can be used to dry the telescope at the end of the cleaning process. When telescopes are frequently autoclaved, a film of deposits may develop on the glass surface over time, due to foreign matter in the steam. This may result in a chemical reaction between the foreign matter and the glass surface. These deposits can be removed using a special cleaning paste, which is also suitable for removing deposits such as disinfectant residues from glass surfaces in general. However, the special cleaning paste should only be used when the image becomes clouded or blurred (after approximately 10–20 sterilizations), and not as a matter of routine after every cleaning.

## Sterilization Procedures

Hopkins telescopes that are marked as autoclavable can be steam-autoclaved using the following procedures.

- Clean and dry the telescope and carefully place it in the sterilization container.
- Autoclave at a maximum temperature of 134° C (272° F) for 5–8 min at 2.2 atmospheric pressures. When the autoclave cycle is completed, remove the container from the autoclave and allow the telescope to cool down to room temperature before removing the top container.
- During steam autoclaving, the telescope should not come into direct contact with metal instruments, trays etc. Any sudden change in temperature may cause the glass component in the telescope to fracture. Exposing the telescope to air immediately after removing it from the autoclave can also cause damage to the telescope. In addition, forced cooling by pouring cool sterile liquid over the telescope must be avoided.

## ■ Minimally Invasive Neuro-Otological Surgery

The introduction of new technologies in many fields, including anesthesia, imaging, diagnosis, micro-instrumentation, neural monitoring, lasers, and endoscopy, has led to tremendous advances in the otoneurosurgery in the cerebellopontine angle is that it allows this deep and delicate area to be reached with minimal morbidity, and provides more comprehensive mapping of the neurovascular components running through it.

Endoscopy is one aspect of the approach involved in minimally invasive surgery—the term referring to new surgical approaches that attempt to minimize skin incisions, bone exposure, and harmful retraction of neural tissue, which has also been described as the "keyhole approach." The underlying assumption is not that "smaller is better," but that "smaller is safer."

Minimally invasive surgery must satisfy five distinct criteria (Gerszten et al. 1995):

1 The technique must be less invasive than currently used techniques, while maintaining safety.
2 The efficacy of the technique should be similar to or better than that of standard techniques.
3 The technique should lead to a shorter recovery time for the patient, both in terms of the length of hospital stay and in the time required to resume daily tasks.
4 The technique must be more cost-effective.
5 The technique must be technically feasible for the majority of surgeons, both in terms of the level of surgical skill required and with regard to the availability of affordable new equipment.

In addition, minimally invasive otoneurosurgery aims to achieve acceptance as the new current standard of care.

## The Keyhole Retrosigmoid Approach

The minimal retrosigmoid approach was first described by Bremond et al. (1974, Bremond and Garcin 1975). The key points of the technique are as follows (O'Donoghue et al. 1994):

- The patient is placed in the supine position on the operating table, with the head turned so that the involved side is uppermost. The surgeon remains in the usual otologic position.
- With the patient under endotracheal anesthesia, a 7-cm incision is made along the posterior margin of the mastoid process. The skin and soft tissue are elevated from the posterior margin of the mastoid process and adjacent suboccipital region, and held in place using a self-retaining retractor. The mastoid emissary vein is the surgical landmark on which to center the retromastoid craniotomy.
- The craniotomy consists of a 1.5-cm circular trephine behind and close to the sigmoid sinus. The dura is opened, and cerebrospinal fluid is allowed to drain freely for several minutes.
- The cerebellum retracts spontaneously due to profound balanced anesthesia including a narcotic (propofol) and an analgesic (Sulfentanil); this is combined with assisted hyperventilation, resulting in hypocapnia ($P_{CO_2}$ 25 mmHg). We never use a retractor in the cerebellum. We protect the surface of the cerebellum with Cottonoids in order to obtain a safe corridor within which to operate.
- Under the operating microscope, we start by opening the arachnoid surrounding the acousticofacial nerve-bundle. The cerebrospinal fluid escapes, and the cerebellum spontaneously falls away without the need for retraction.
- At this time, the endoscope is inserted between the posterior wall of the petrous bone and the cerebellum. To maintain aseptic conditions, the surgeon must check the progression of the endoscope using a video camera and monitor (not direct inspection through the eyepiece).

## Micro-Instrumentation

Conventional otology instruments are too short, and the usual neurosurgical instruments are too bulky. Specially adapted instruments with a bayonet handle have been introduced. These facilitate visualization when using the keyhole approach. Each instrument is designed for use in a specific direction (up, down, right, left).

## Nerve Monitoring

Facial nerve monitoring is routinely used. Using two-channel electromyography (EMG) (e.g., Nim 2 or Neurosign), spontaneous EMG is continuously monitored to detect changes in activity related to surgery.

Professional personnel are needed for the use of multichannel EMG (e.g., Saphir or Viking IV), with multiple independent functions and simultaneous EMG and evoked auditory potential monitoring.

Intraoperative cochlear nerve action potential recording is carried out during microvascular decompression and in attempts at hearing preservation with small or medium-sized acoustic neuroma tumors. The placement of the intraoperative recording electrode is the most technically difficult part of the procedure.

## Endoscopes

We recommend rigid instruments for precise surgical maneuvers. The safest endoscope is 6 cm in length and 4 mm in diameter, with a 0° angle. This provides a panoramic view, and the limited length prevents inadvertent contact with deeper-lying structures. Other useful endoscopes are 11 cm in length, 4 mm and 2.7 mm in diameter, with 0° and 30° angles.

The 60° and 70° angled endoscopes are dangerous, since the surgeon cannot appreciate the exact position of the tip of the endoscope.

## References

Bremond G, Garcin M, Magnan J, Bonnaud G. L'abord à minima de l'espace ponto-cérébelleux. Cah ORL 1974; 19: 443–60.

Bremond G, Garcin M. Microsurgical approach to the cerebellopontine angle. J Laryngol 1975; 89: 237–48.

Doyen E. Retro-Gasserian neurotomy of the trigeminal nerve, with the aid of intracranial endoscopy. In: Doyen E. Surgical therapeutics and operative techniques, vol. 1. London: Baillière, Tindall, Cox, 1917: 599–602.

Gerszten P, Clyde B, McLaughin M, Jho H. Criteria on which to judge all minimally invasive neurosurgical techniques. Pittsburgh: Joint International Congress on Minimally Invasive Techniques in Neurosurgery and Otolaryngology, 1995.

McKennan K. Endoscopy of the internal auditory canal during hearing conservation acoustic tumor surgery Am J Otol 1993; 14: 259–62.

Magnan J, Chays A, Caces F, et al. Apport de l'endoscopie de l'angle ponto-cérébelleux par voie rétro-sigmoïde. Ann Otolaryngol Chir Cervicofac 1993; 110: 259–65.

Magnan J, Chays A, Lepetre C, Pencroffi E. Surgical perspectives on endoscopy of the cerebellopontine angle. Am J Otol 1994; 15: 366–70.

O'Donoghue G, Greengrass S, Magnan J. Endoscopy in otology and otoneurosurgery. Adv Otolaryngol Head Neck Surg 1994; 8: 43–67.

O'Donoghue GM, O'Flynn P. Endoscopic anatomy of the cerebellopontine angle. Am J Otol 1993; 14: 122–5.

Oppel F, Mulch G. Selective trigeminal root section via an endoscopic transpyramidal retrolabyrinthine approach. Acta Neurochir 1979; 28 (Suppl): 565–71.

Prott W. Möglichkeiten einer Endoskopie des Kleinhirnbrückwinkels auf transpyramidalem-retrolabyrinthärem Zugangsweg: Cisternoscopie. HNO 1974; 22: 337–41.

# 2 Endoscopic Anatomy of the Cerebellopontine Angle and Adjacent Structures

## ▣ Posterior View of the Cerebellopontine Angle (Figs. 8–10)

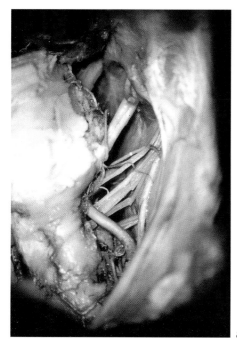

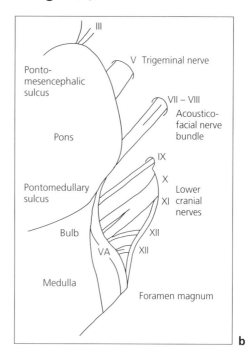

Fig. **8a, b** The petrosal or anterior surface of the cerebellum faces the posterior surface of the temporal bone and the brain stem. The neurovascular bundles define four levels from superior to inferior: trigeminal, acousticofacial, lower cranial, and foramen magnum.

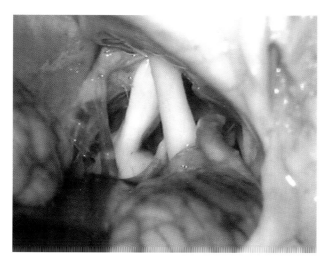

Fig. **9** Right retrosigmoid approach under the operating microscope. The acousticofacial nerve bundle crosses the middle of the cerebellopontine angle (CPA). Its entrance into the porus acusticus provides an unquestionable identification. The flocculus overlies the root entry zone of the cochleovestibular and facial nerves. Superiorly, the trigeminal nerve exits the pons and travels obliquely in an anterosuperior direction toward the petrous apex. Inferiorly, the posterior inferior cerebellar artery and the glossopharyngeal nerve are seen.

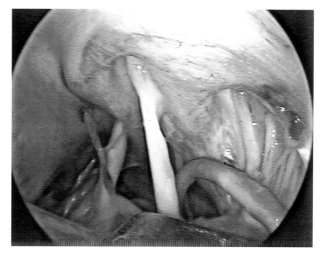

Fig. **10** Right retrosigmoid approach: endoscopic view of the CPA. The acousticofacial nerve bundle is the reference level. Superior and anterior to the vestibulocochlear nerve lies the trigeminal area, which consists of the superior petrosal vein, the trigeminal nerve, and the superior cerebellar artery. Inferior and posterior to the vestibulocochlear nerve lies the lower cranial nerve area, which consists of the posterior inferior cerebellar artery and the glossopharyngeal, vagus, and accessory nerves. Using a 0° endoscope, the points of entry of the nerves into the temporal bone are clearly seen.

## Trigeminal Area (Figs. 11–19)

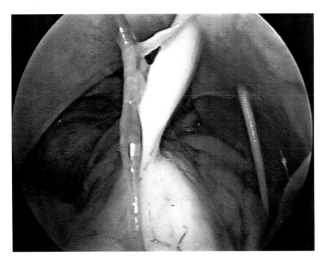

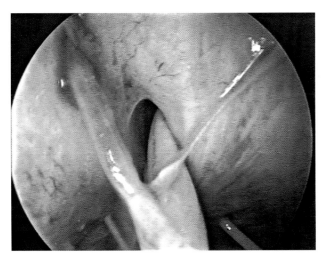

Fig. **11**  The trigeminal nerve from the porus to the Meckel cavity (trigeminal cavity). Posterior to the trigeminal nerve lies the superior petrosal vein (Dandy vein). Superior to the trigeminal nerve the superior cerebellar artery. In the background and inferiorly, the abducent nerve and basilar artery are seen. In the background and superiorly, the free border of the tentorium and the mesencephalic area are seen.

Fig. **12**  The entrance of the trigeminal nerve into the Meckel cavity. The superior petrosal vein prior to its entrance into the superior petrosal sinus is seen.

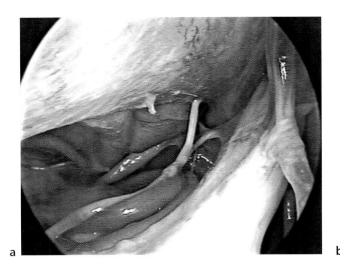

a

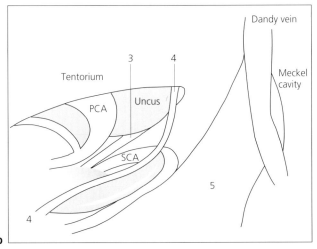

b

Fig. **13a, b**  Here, the tip of the endoscope is positioned at the level of the posterior margin of the trigeminal nerve in order to carry out an inspection above it, visualizing the rostral and cranial branches of the superior cerebellar artery and the trochlear nerve. The trochlear nerve disappears under the free margin of the tentorium. The point of entrance is just before the cavernous sinus. In the background, the oculomotor nerve and the posterior cerebral artery, are seen, as well as the free border of the tentorium and the uncus of the temporal lobe.

3    Oculomotor nerve
4    Trochlear nerve
5    Trigeminal nerve
PCA  Posterior cerebral artery
SCA  Superior cerebellar artery

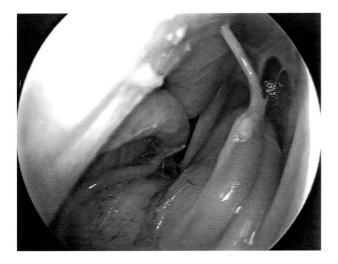

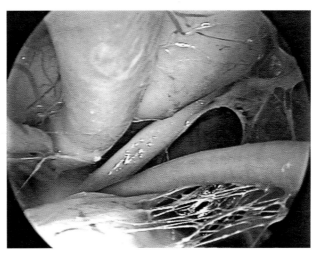

Fig. **14** The endoscope is positioned between the trigeminal nerve and the tentorium. The superior cerebellar artery encircles the brain stem above the trigeminal nerve and below the trochlear nerve. The superior cerebellar artery, arising as a single trunk, bifurcates into rostral and caudal trunks. The pontomesencephalic incisure, with the third cranial nerve, lies between the uncus and the trochlear nerve. The posterior cerebral artery and a branch passing to the mesencephalon are seen.

Fig. **15** Arterial relationships around the oculomotor nerve. The superior cerebellar artery lies inferiorly, and the posterior cerebral artery superiorly. The exit zone of the third cranial nerve between the superior cerebellar artery and the posterior cerebral artery is seen.

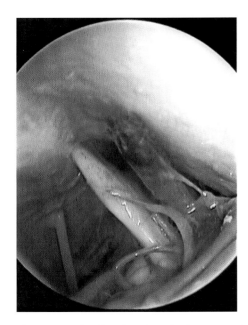

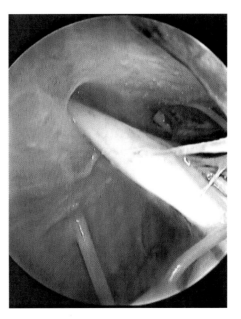

Fig. **16** Left side. The trigeminal nerve and Dandy vein are seen entering the superior petrosal sinus.

Fig. **17** The trigeminal nerve exits the posterior fossa to enter the middle cranial fossa, passing forward beneath the tentorial attachment to enter the Meckel cavity. The Dandy vein lies superiorly. Inferiorly, the abducent nerve enters the Dorello canal.

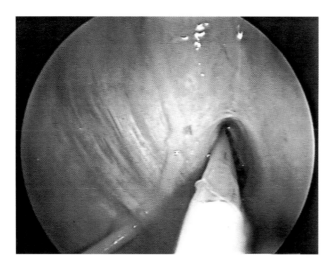

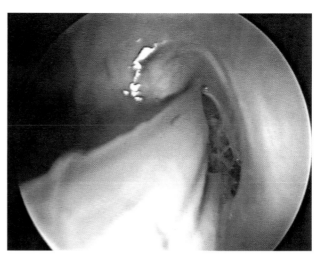

Fig. **18**   Using the 30° angled endoscope, the Meckel cavity and the intradural course of the abducent nerve are seen, delimiting the petroclival area. After piercing the inner layer of the dura mater, the nerve changes direction and courses medially toward the petrous apex.

Fig. **19**   The major sensory root and the minor motor root within the Meckel cavity. This close-up view allows visualization of the roof and the bifurcation at the bottom of the Meckel cavity.

## Acousticofacial Nerve Bundle (Figs. 20, 21)

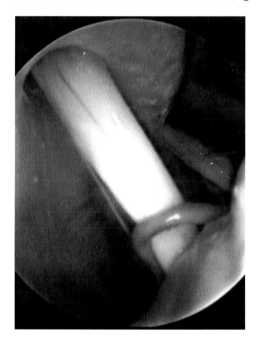 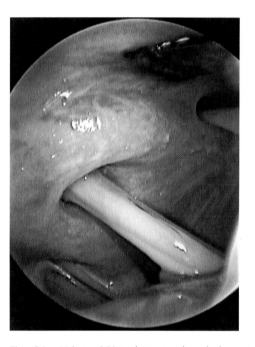

Fig. **20** Left side. The acousticofacial nerve bundle runs obliquely from the pons to the internal acoustic meatus in a superolateral direction. Its length between the entry zone of the nerves and the porus of the internal acoustic meatus varies from 8 mm to 14 mm. A groove or raphe on the posterior surface of the cochleovestibular nerves indicates the division of the cochlear segment inferiorly and the vestibular segment superiorly. A labyrinthine artery arises from the loop of the anterior inferior cerebellar artery. The fifth nerve lies in the background.

Fig. **21** Using a 30° endoscope, the whole posterior surface of the petrous bone is visualized. The internal auditory meatus lies approximately at the center. The acousticofacial nerve bundle consists of the eighth cranial nerve (vestibulocochlear) and seventh (facial). The eighth nerve is divided into two components, the cochlear nerve inferiorly and the vestibular nerve superiorly. The facial nerve runs parallel and anterior to the vestibulocochlear nerve.

## Lower Cranial Nerve Area (Figs. 22–24)

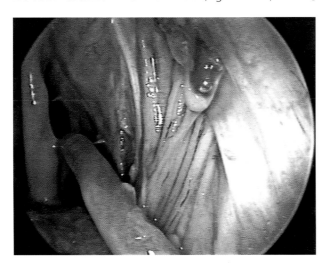

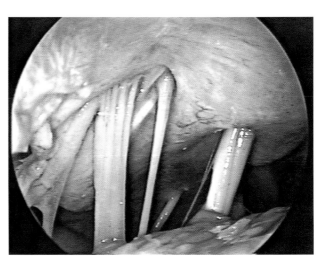

Fig. **22**   Right side. The acousticofacial nerve bundle, posterior inferior cerebellar artery, and lower cranial nerves are seen in the lower part. The inferior cerebellar vein (not constant) enters the jugular bulb. As the posterior fossa is approached from behind the sigmoid sinus, the jugular dural fold appears as a white linear structure overlying the lower cranial nerves.

Fig. **23**   Left side. The 30° angled endoscope provides an overview of the inferior part of the CPA. On the right lies the acousticofacial nerve bundle, with the anterior inferior cerebellar artery; the glossopharyngeal nerve and the vagus nerve, as multiple filaments, form three to five major nerve bundles and the accessory nerve.

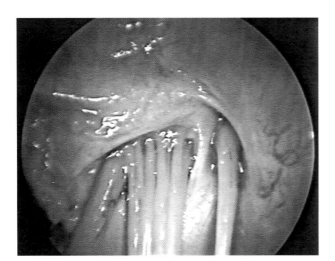

Fig. **24**   A closer view of the pars nervosa of the jugular foramen. The glossopharyngeal nerve has its own dural porus, which is situated 0–3 mm upwards from the dural porus of the tenth cranial nerve. The vagus and the accessory nerve exit the posterior fossa together in a sleeve of dura through the jugular foramen.

## Foramen Magnum (Figs. 25–36)

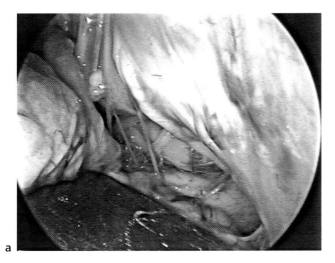

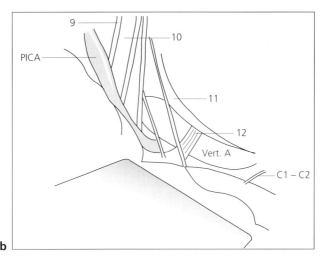

Fig. **25a, b**   The right side of the bulbomedullary junction. It is the lowermost and narrowest part of the posterior fossa. This area requires special dissection prior to endoscopic investigation between the pontomedullary stem and the jugular foramen.

| 9 | Glossopharyngeal nerve |
|---|---|
| 10 | Vagus nerve |
| 11 | Accessory nerve |
| 12 | Hypoglossal nerve |
| PICA | Posterior inferior cerebellar artery |
| Vert. A | Vertebral artery |

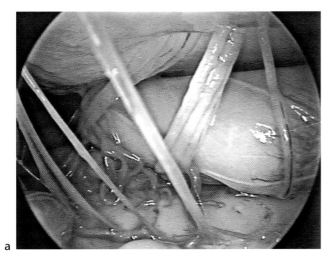

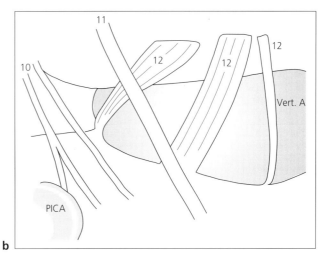

Fig. **26a, b**   Right side. The root fibers of the hypoglossal nerve (12) collect in two bundles, which pierce the dura in two dural pori. The hypoglossal nerve is situated more anteriorly and medially than the root fibers of the lower cranial nerves. The arterial relationship is the vertebral artery, with perforating arteries to the brain stem. The curved vertebral artery displaces and stretches the hypoglossal nerve fibers.

| 10 | Vagus nerve |
|---|---|
| 11 | Accessory nerve |
| 12 | Hypoglossal nerve |
| PICA | Posterior inferior cerebellar artery |
| Vert. A | Vertebral artery |

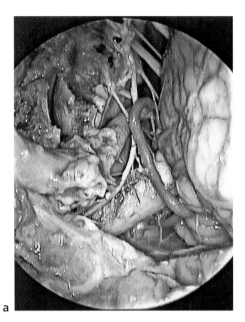

a

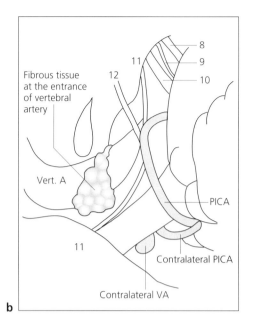

b

Fig. **27a, b**   Left side. Combined transsigmoid, suboccipital and extreme lateral approaches provide an overview off the craniocervical junction, the foramen magnum area, and the surrounding structures of the medullary stem.

| 8 | Vestibulocochlear nerve |
|---|---|
| 9 | Glossopharyngeal nerve |
| 10 | Vagus nerve |
| 11 | Accessory nerve |
| 12 | Hypoglossal nerve |
| PICA | Posterior inferior cerebellar artery |
| VA | Vertebral artery |

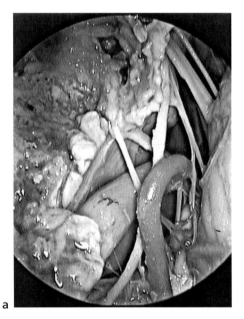

a

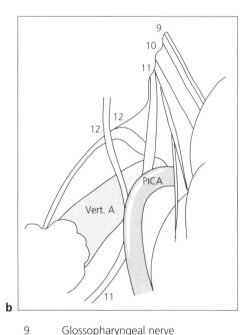

b

Fig. **28a, b**   The posterior inferior cerebellar artery travels through the nerve fiber roots of the accessory nerve and encircles the brain stem. The course of the vertebral artery is inferior and anterior to the lower cranial nerves and the hypoglossal nerve. Fibrous tissue surrounds the entrance of the vertebral artery into the CPA.

| 9 | Glossopharyngeal nerve |
|---|---|
| 10 | Vagus nerve |
| 11 | Accessory nerve |
| 12 | Hypoglossal nerve |
| PICA | Posterior inferior cerebellar artery |
| Vert. A | Vertebral artery |

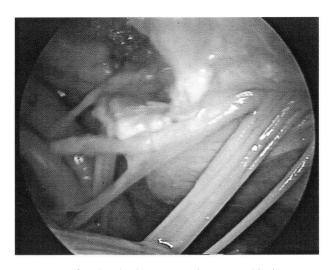

Fig. **29** Left side. The lower cranial nerves, with the posterior inferior cerebellar artery arising from the vertebral artery in the background.

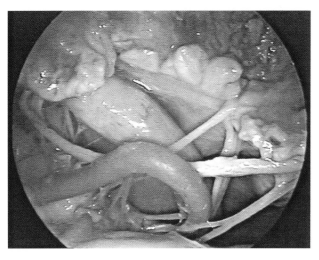

Fig. **30** Neurovascular relationships between the exit zone of the root fiber bundles of the eleventh and twelfth nerves, the posterior inferior cerebellar and vertebral arteries. Fibrous tissue is seen around the vertebral artery.

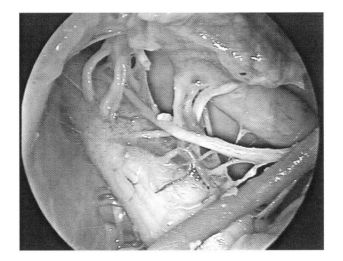

Fig. **31** The root fibers of the spinal accessory nerve and the fibers of C1 and C2. The entrance of the vertebral artery is the boundary between the foramen magnum and the spinal part of the accessory nerve.

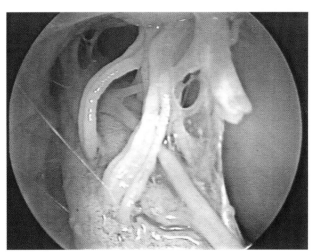

Fig. **32** A 30° endoscope provides an overview of the medullary canal.

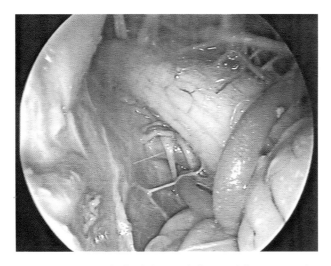

Fig. **33**   Two cerebellar lobes and the medullary stem. The posterior inferior cerebellar artery encircles the medullary stem. The opposite vertebral artery exits from the dural porus and raises the hypoglossal nerve.

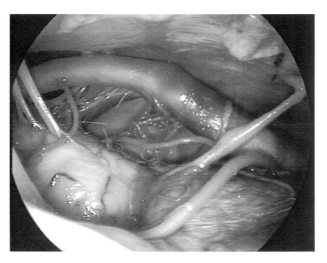

Fig. **34**   The pontomedullary junction. The vertebral artery junction is at the level of the junction of the inferior and mid-clivus. The basilar artery runs in a straight line on the surface of the pons. The exit zones of the hypoglossal and abducent nerves are at the same level. The abducent nerve exits from the pontomedullary junction, and ascends in a rostral and lateral direction toward the clivus.

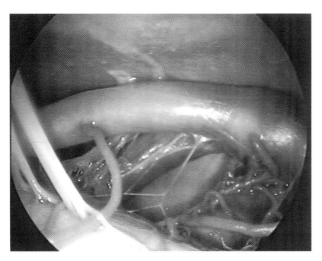

Fig. **35**   A closer view of the anterior border of the pontomedullary stem and the vertebral artery junction and origin of the basilar artery. Perforating arteries arise from the vertebral and basilar arteries.

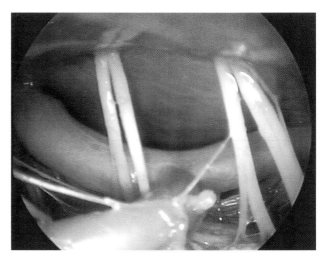

Fig. **36**   The endoscope is focusing on the hypoglossal nerve area. The posterior inferior cerebellar artery arises from the vertebral artery in the background, and runs between the two bundles of the hypoglossal nerve.

# Superior View of the Cerebellopontine Angle (Figs. 37–39)

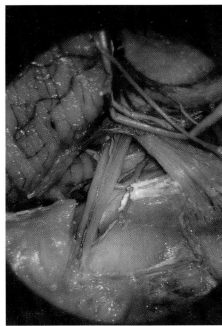

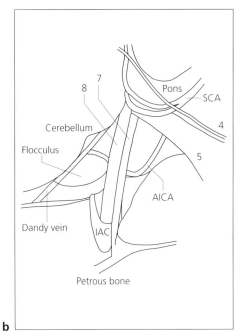

a

b

Fig. **37a, b** Anteriorly and superiorly lie the trigeminal nerve and the superior cerebellar artery. Posteriorly and inferiorly, the acousticofacial nerve bundle and the anterior inferior cerebellar artery are seen.

4      Trochlear nerve
5      Trigeminal nerve
7      Facial nerve
8      Vestibulocochlear nerve
AICA   Anterior inferior cerebellar artery
IAC    Internal auditory canal
SCA    Superior cerebellar artery

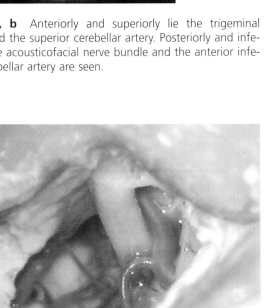

Fig. **38**   Right enlarged middle fossa approach. The internal auditory canal has been opened, revealing the acousticofacial nerve bundle contained within it. The facial nerve runs anteriorly, and the superior vestibular nerve lies posteriorly. The loop of the anterior inferior cerebellar artery runs near the meatus, below the acousticofacial nerve bundle.

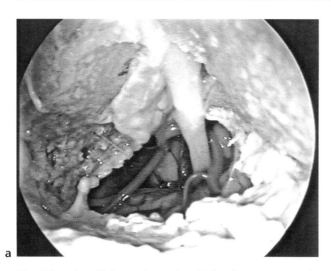

a

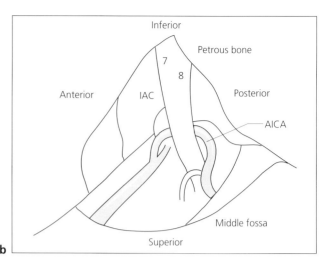

b

Fig. **39a, b** Right enlarged middle fossa approach. Endoscopic view of the acousticofacial nerve bundle in the internal auditory canal and in the cerebellopontine angle.

| | |
|---|---|
| 7 | Facial nerve |
| 8 | Vestibulocochlear nerve |
| AICA | Anterior inferior cerebellar artery |
| IAC | Internal auditory canal |

## Intracanalicular Part of the Acousticofacial Nerve Bundle (Figs. 40–42)

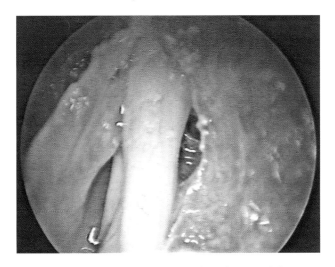

Fig. **40**   A closer view at the level of the fundus of the internal auditory canal. The facial nerve lies anteriorly and superiorly. The vestibular nerve posteriorly is separated from the facial nerve by a plane of cleavage. The cochlear nerve is located inferior to the facial nerve.

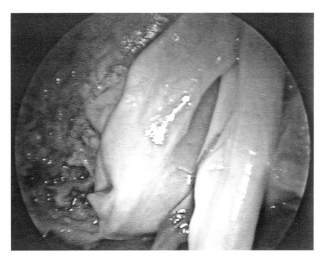

Fig. **41**   The cochlear nerve travels along an inferior course in the internal auditory canal. Inferior to the vestibular nerve at the porus acusticus, it becomes inferior to the facial nerve at the lateral end of the internal auditory canal. There is a labyrinthine artery coursing between the cochlear and facial nerves.

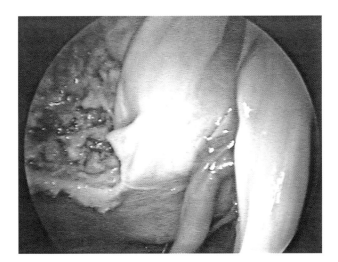

Fig. **42**   A closer view at the level of the porus acusticus. The anterior inferior cerebellar artery forms a vascular loop and gives off labyrinthine arteries, which fix the contact between the artery and the inferior surface of the acousticofacial nerve bundle at the inferior lip of the meatus.

## Cerebellopontine Part of the
## Acousticofacial Nerve Bundle (Figs. 43–46)

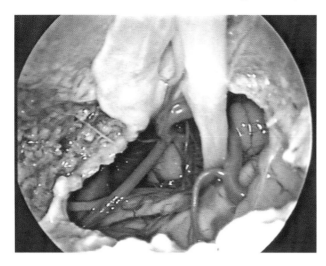

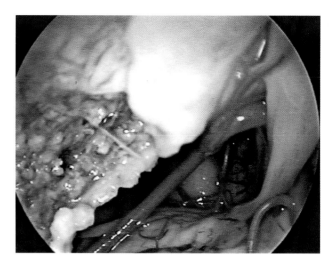

Fig. **43** The acousticofacial nerve bundle exits from the pons, and travels obliquely in the CPA in a superolateral direction towards the internal auditory canal. The facial nerve exits immediately anterior to the roots of the cochlear and vestibular nerves. The relationships with the anterior inferior cerebellar artery are clearly identified.

Fig. **44** The anterior inferior cerebellar artery and the root exit zone of the facial nerve are exposed.

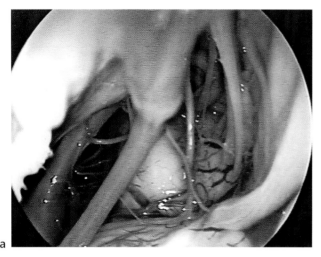

a

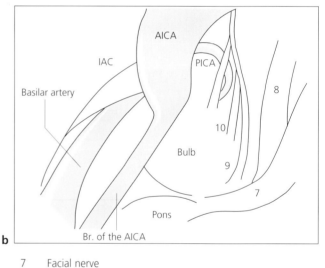

b

Fig. **45a, b** The root exit zone of the facial nerve is anterior to the root of the cochlear nerve and superior to the rootlets of the lower cranial nerves.

| | |
|---|---|
| 7 | Facial nerve |
| 8 | Vestibulocochlear nerve |
| 9 | Glossopharyngeal nerve |
| 10 | Vagus nerve |
| AICA | Anterior inferior cerebellar artery |
| IAC | Internal auditory canal |
| PICA | Posterior inferior cerebellar artery |

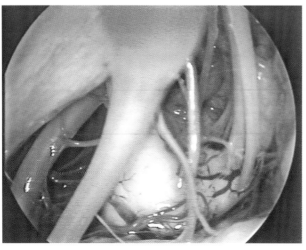

Fig. **46** The pontobulbar junction and the roots of the lower cranial nerves are visualized. The loop of the posterior inferior cerebellar artery is seen in the background.

# Anterior to the Acousticofacial Nerve
## Bundle (Figs. 47–50)

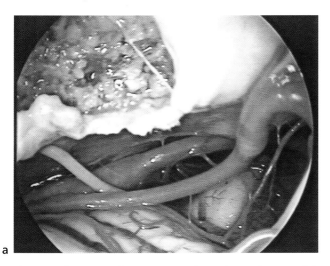

a

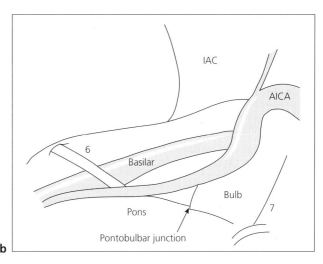

b

Fig. **47a, b**   From the porus acusticus, the endoscope follows the course of the anterior inferior cerebellar artery in order to reach the anterior part the cerebellopontine angle and the trigeminal area.

6       Abducent nerve
7       Facial nerve
AICA   Anterior inferior cerebellar artery
IAC    Internal auditory canal

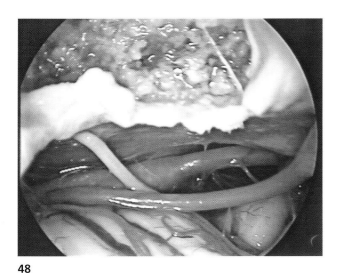

48

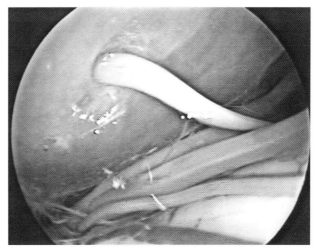

49

Fig. **48**   The abducent nerve. In the background, the vertebral and basilar arteries are first visualized. The origin of the anterior inferior cerebellar artery is clearly seen.

Fig. **49**   The abducent nerve enters its dural porus, Dorello's canal. The anterior inferior cerebellar artery arises from the basilar artery.

Fig. **50**   Using a 30° endoscope, the trigeminal area is visualized superior to the abducent nerve, and the trigeminal trunk is visualized from the pons to the petrous apex. Motor and sensory roots are identified.

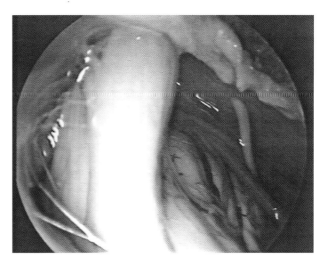

50

## Inferior to the Acousticofacial Nerve
## Bundle (Figs. 51–54)

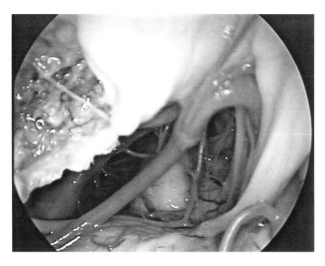

Fig. **51**   A closer view of the CPA from the porus acusticus. The root exit zones of the facial nerve and the abducent nerve are seen. Note the relationships between the loop of the anterior inferior cerebellar artery and the acousticofacial nerve bundle. The lower cranial nerves are seen in the background.

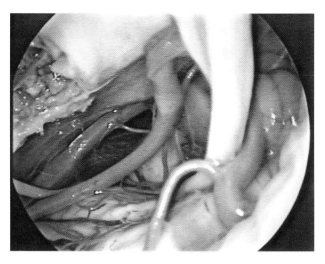

Fig. **52**   A deeper view, showing the relationships between the vertebral artery and the lower clivus; the flocculus lobe and the anterior inferior cerebellar artery are seen.

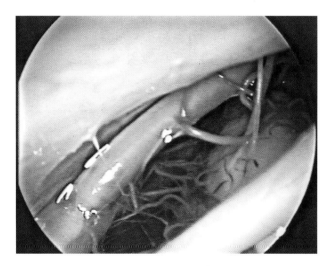

Fig. **53**   The vertebral artery joins its fellow on the opposite side and gives off several perforating arteries to the spinal cord.

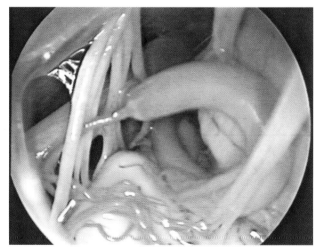

Fig. **54**   The tip of the endoscope lies between the acousticofacial nerve bundle and the anterior inferior cerebellar artery. The posterior inferior cerebellar artery arises from the vertebral artery, runs between the root fibers of the hypoglossal nerve, and forms a loop below the roots of the lower cranial nerves, before coursing in a posterior direction.

# References

Barrow D. Surgery of the cranial nerves of the posterior fossa. Park Ridge, Illinois: American Association of Neurological Surgeons, 1993.

Kim HN, Kim YH, Park Y, Kim GR. Variability of the surgical anatomy of the neurovascular complex of the cerebellopontine angle. Ann Otol Rhinol Laryngol 1990; 99: 288–96.

Lang J. Anatomy of the brain stem and the lower cranial nerves, vessels and surrounding structures. Am J Otol 1985; 6 (Suppl): 1–19.

Perneczky A, Tschabitscher M, Resch K. Endoscopic anatomy for neurosurgery. Stuttgart: Thieme, 1994.

Sanna M, Saleh E, Russo A, Taibah A. Atlas of temporal bone and lateral skull base surgery. Stuttgart: Thieme, 1995.

Silverstein H, Willcox T, Rosenberg S, Seidman M. The jugular dural fold: a helpful skull base landmark to the cranial nerves. Skull Base Surg 1995; 5: 57–61.

# 3 Microscopic and Endoscopic Neuro-Otological Surgery

## ■ Incapacitating Vertigo

### Ménière Disease

Endoscopic section of the vestibular nerve using a retrolabyrinthine approach was proposed by Oppel and Handrock in 1984. More recently, Loh (1995) demonstrated that it is possible to use both endoscopic and laser techniques to carry out vestibular neurotomy. Since 1974, we have carried out vestibular neurotomy via a retrosigmoid approach, which in our experience provides the best and easiest view of the acousticofacial nerve bundle, with a very low complication rate.

Endoscopic vestibular neurotomy can be performed using a similar approach, and since 1993 we have been developing this minimally invasive technique. We have been able to carry out vestibular neurotomy with the endoscope alone in 16 of 45 patients undergoing vestibular neurotomy to control disabling vertigo in Ménière's disease. Difficulties and obstacles encountered during endoscopic vestibular neurotomy included:

– Insufficient spontaneous retraction of the cerebellum prior to opening of the basal cisterns.
– The presence of thick arachnoid wrapping, requiring dissection.
– The presence of a vascular loop hindering direct access to the acousticofacial nerve bundle.
– Difficulty in determining with certainty whether the nerve section is complete.

Refinements in the instruments available are necessary to overcome these difficulties. As yet, there are no advantages for the use of endoscopic vestibular neurotomy in comparison with the operating microscope with regard to the safety and efficiency of the operation. Less time is required for the procedure using the operating microscope.

### Retrosigmoid Approach

The following presentation illustrates the view obtained under an operating microscope and with the endoscope during vestibular neurotomy via the retrosigmoid approach.

## Exposure of the Acousticofacial Nerve Bundle (Figs. 55, 56)

## Intervestibulocochlear Cleavage Plane (Fig. 57)

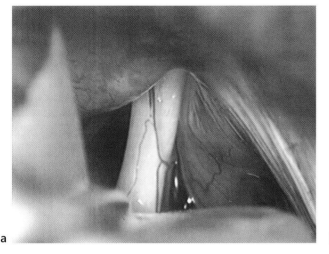

a

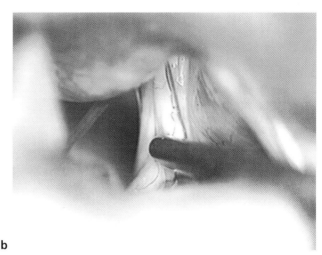

b

Fig. **55a, b**   Microscopic right vestibular neurotomy. The auditory nerve hides the facial nerve, which runs anteriorly.

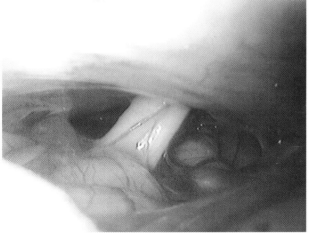

a

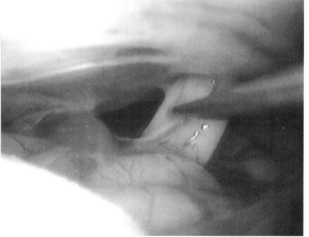

b

Fig. **56a, b**   Endoscopic left vestibular neurotomy.

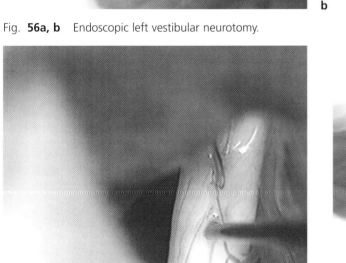

a

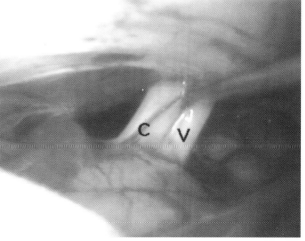

b

Fig. **57   a** Operative microscope (right side); **b** endoscope (left side). If at first sight it seems impossible to identify and separate the vestibular nerve (V) from the cochlear nerve (C), a small dissector can be used to locate the groove that marks the cleavage plane along the eighth nerve.

## Identification of the Vestibular Nerve

The vestibular fibers are more superior (rostral) and closest to the fifth cranial nerve. The cochlear nerve is inferior (caudal) and closest to the ninth nerve.

## Section of the Vestibular Nerve

Vestibular neurotomy is performed with microsurgical scissors (Figs. **58a**, **59a**). After complete neurotomy, the ends of the nerve retract spontaneously. The facial nerve, which is much deeper, is safe from injury (Figs. **58**, **59**).

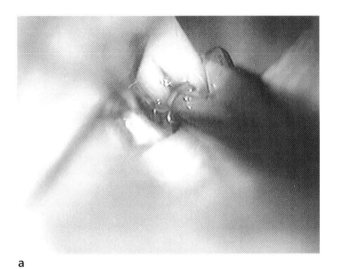

a

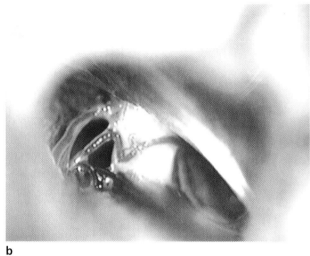

b

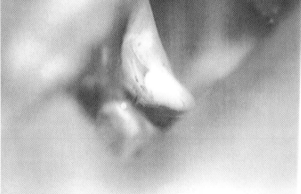

c

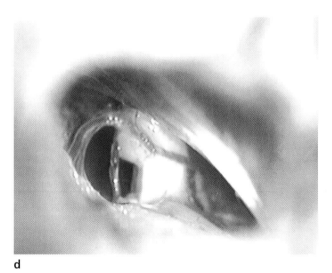

d

Fig. **58a–e**   Under the operating microscope. **a**, **c** Left side. **b**, **d**, **e** Right side.

c  Cochlear nerve
f  Facial nerve
v  Vestibular nerve

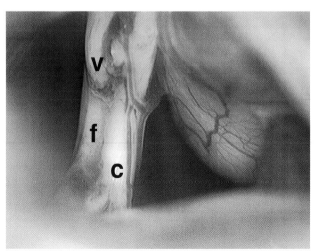

e

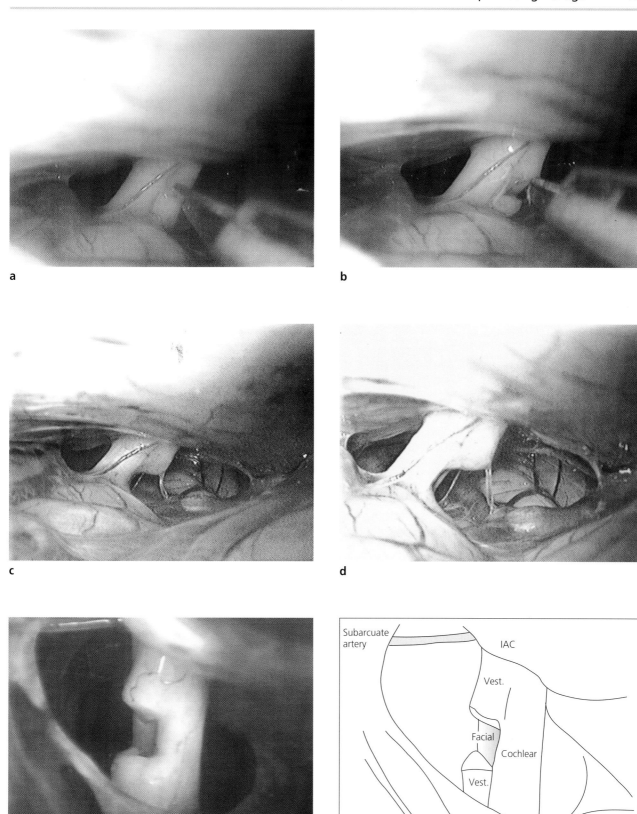

Fig. **59a–f**   Endoscopic vestibular neurotomy. **a**, **b**, **c**, **d** Left side. **e**, **f** Right side.

IAC  Internal auditory canal

The basic effect of vestibular neurotomy is to allow vestibular compensation to take place, suppressing both vertigo and associated symptoms. This functional recovery of balance and oculomotor function through central sensory substitution requires a regeneration of neuronal activity in vestibular nuclei from which the afferent path has been disconnected. The vestibular nuclei speed up thanks to connections with the opposite vestibular nuclei and with the proprioceptive and visual systems. This neurological phenomenon restores a new balance at the level of the vestibular nuclei, and reduces the risk of Ménière's disease becoming bilateral.

In our experience in 195 retrosigmoid vestibular neurotomies, surgical management of incapacitating Ménière's disease is not only an effective way of controlling incapacitating vertigo, but also the best way of preserving hearing in the long term. These findings suggest that surgery should be carried out at an early stage of Ménière's disease in order to preserve hearing in the affected ear.

## Retrolabyrinthine Approach (Figs. 60–65)

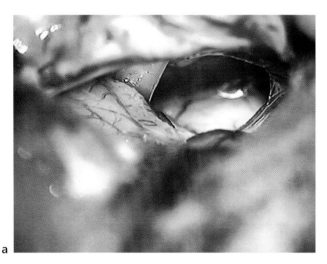

a

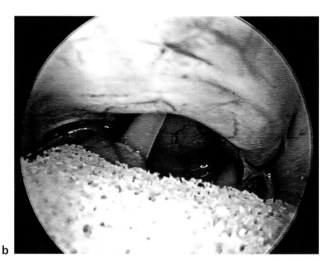

b

Fig. **60a, b**  A left retrolabyrinthine approach view through the operating microscope (**a**) and through a straight-viewing endoscope, diameter 4 mm (**b**). The anterior position of the sigmoid sinus reduces the size of the retrolabyrinthine approach.

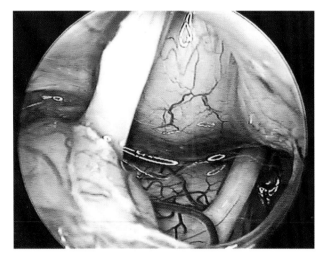

Fig. **61**  Endoscopy is used before the nerve is cut, in order to locate the precise positions of the facial nerve and the vascular loop from the anterior inferior cerebellar artery, or the artery itself. This is particularly important when the floccular lobe is prominent, covering the medial end of the acoustico-facial nerve bundle, or when the posterior wall of the petrous bone is prominent, concealing the entrance of the nerve into the porus acusticus.

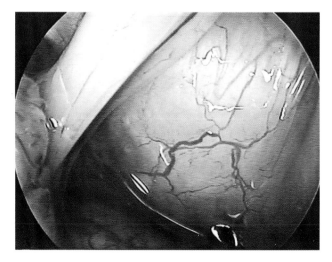

Fig. **62**  Using a 30° angled endoscope, the root of the facial nerve is seen anteriorly, and the cleavage plane between the eighth and seventh nerves is visualized.

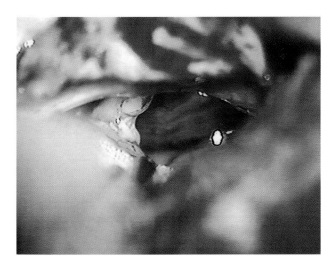

Fig. **63**   Again, endoscopy is used after vestibular neurotomy in order to confirm the completeness of the section.

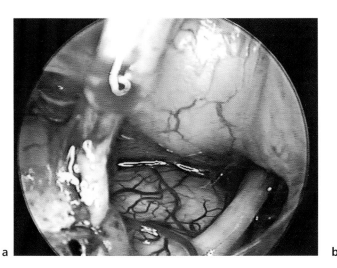

a

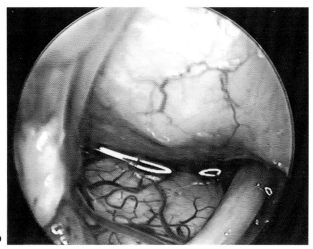

b

Fig. **64a, b**   Initially, some fibers are still present, and a vascular loop from the anterior inferior cerebellar artery is intimately attached to the remaining fibers between the cochlear and facial nerves. This gives the surgeon more detailed knowledge of the relationships between vessels and nerves, and consequently leads to safer surgery.

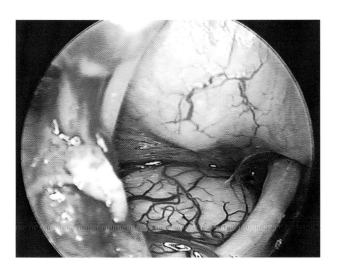

Fig. **65**   The second endoscopic check clearly demonstrates complete section of the vestibular nerve, preservation of the vascular loop, and the integrity of the cochlear and facial nerves.

## Disabling Positional Vertigo

Microvascular decompression of the eighth cranial nerve for the treatment of vertigo has not met with the same degree of acceptance as in treatment for trigeminal neuralgia and hemifacial spasm (Bergsneider and Becker 1995). Reservations regarding the procedure have centered on two main issues. Firstly, the confusing description of the symptom makes reliable diagnosis difficult. Disabling positional vertigo as defined by Moller (1991, Jannetta et al. 1984) is not a clear entity. However, abnormal brain stem auditory evoked potential latencies, in association with vascular compression of the auditory nerve identified on magnetic resonance imaging (MRI), appear to be regarded as sufficient grounds for surgical intervention. Secondly, the difficulty or even impossibility of mobilizing the vascular loop, when the loop of the anterior inferior cerebellar artery lies between or around the acousticofacial nerve, reduces the efficacy of neurovascular decompression.

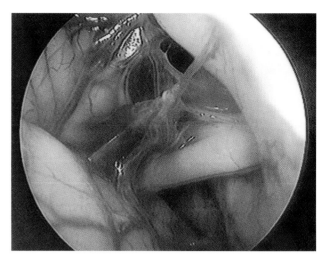

Fig. **66**  Endoscopic view of the course of the loop of the anterior inferior cerebellar artery between the eighth and seventh nerves, and the subarcuate artery at the top of the vascular loop.

### First Case  (Figs. **66**, **67**)

A 54-year-old man had been suffering vertigo, which did not respond to medical treatment, for six years. The patient had right sensorineural hearing loss, more marked in the higher frequencies, and right vestibular hypofunction on caloric testing. The MRI showed an anterior inferior cerebellar artery loop compressing the eighth nerve.

### Second Case (Figs. **68–70**)

A 54-year-old woman, who had been suffering disabling positional vertigo and left tinnitus for nine years. The MRI assessment showed an aberrant venous structure adjacent to the acousticofacial nerve bundle, reaching the internal auditory canal, on T1 turboflash imaging. On the T2 constructive interference in steady state (CISS) image sequence, a loop of the anterior inferior cerebellar artery was identified passing between the nerves.

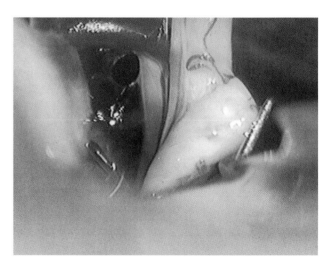

Fig. **67**  As it was impossible to mobilize the vascular loop between the acousticofacial nerves, a vestibular neurotomy was carried out.

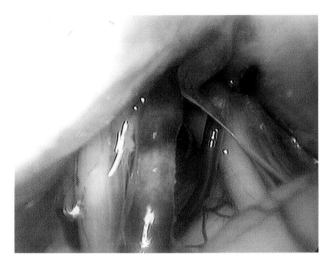

Fig. **68** Endoscopic view of the left cerebellopontine angle using a straight endoscope, diameter 4 mm. The aberrant venous structure lies above the eighth nerve.

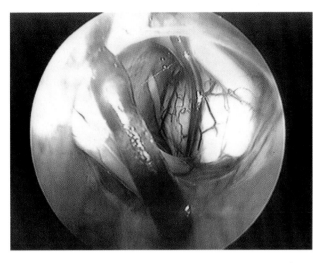

Fig. **69** Using a 30° angled endoscope, the course of the vein is well identified. It arises from the cerebellum and curves through the acoustic meatus toward the superior petrosal sinus.

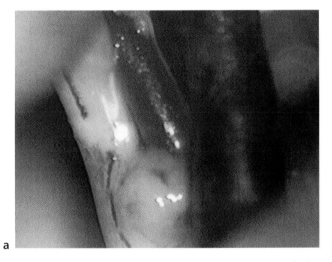

a

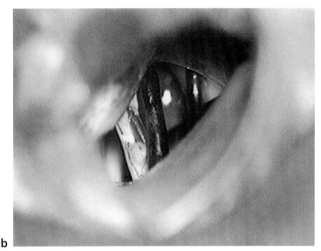

b

Fig. **70a, b** Under the operating microscope, vestibular neurotomy was carried out, exposing the loop of the anterior inferior cerebellar artery.

## References

Bergsneider M, Becker D. Vascular compression syndrome of the vestibular nerve: a critical analysis. Otolaryngol Head Neck Surg 1995; 112: 118–24.

Iurato S, Onofri M. Long-term follow-up after middle fossa vestibular neurectomy for Ménière's disease. ORL J Otorhinolaryngol Relat Spec 1995; 57:141–7.

Jannetta P, Moller M, Moller A. Disabling positional vertigo. N Engl J Med 1984; 310: 1700–5.

Loh KK. Laser-assisted endoscopic vestibular neurotomy. Paper presented at Joint International Congress on Minimally Invasive Techniques in Neurosurgery and Otolaryngology, Pittsburgh, 17–20 June 1995.

McKenna M, Nadol JB Jr, Ojemann RG, Halpin C. Vestibular neurectomy: retrosigmoid-intracanalicular versus retro-labyrinthine approach. Am J Otol 1996; 17: 253–8.

Magnan J. La chirurgie des vertiges. Encyclopedie Medico-Chirurgicale (EMC) (Paris: Elsevier) Oto-Rhino-Laryngologie 1994; 46–045: 15.

Magnan J, Bremond G, Chays A, et al. Vestibular neurotomy by retrosigmoid approach: technique, indications, results. Am J Otol 1991; 12: 101–4.

Magnan J, Chays A, Locatelli P, et al. Hearing results in Ménière's disease following retrosigmoid vestibular neuroto-my. In: Filipo R, Barbara B, eds. Ménière's disease: perspectives in the 90s. Amsterdam: Kugler, 1994: 565–9.

Moller M. Vascular compression of the eighth cranial nerve as a cause of vertigo. Keio J Med 1991; 40: 146–50.

Oppel F, Handrock M. Endoscopic section of the vestibular nerve by transpyramidal retrolabyrinthine approach in Ménière's disease. Adv Oto-Rhino-Laryngol 1984; 34: 234–41.

Prades JM, Martin C, Chelikh L, Merzougui N. Voie d'abord retrolabyrinthique "optimisée". Interêt dans l'endoscopie de l'angle ponto-cerebelleux. Ann Otolaryngol Chir Cervicofac 1995; 112: 46–51.

Silverstein H, Wanamaker H, Flanzer J, Rosenberg S. Vestibular neurectomy in the United States–1990. Am J Otol 1992, 13: 23–30.

## Hemifacial Spasm

Hemifacial spasm is a troublesome and disabling disease, consisting of a unilateral progressive spasm starting in the orbicularis oculi muscle and gradually spreading down the side of the face. Gardner (1960) was the first to identify an artery–nerve compression in the cerebellopontine angle as explaining the pathogenesis of hemifacial spasm. During the 1970s, Jannetta promoted the use of microvascular decompression as a treatment for hemifacial spasm.

**Pathophysiology.** The vascular loop compression is at the root exit zone of the facial nerve, at the myelin transition zone from the central nervous system to the peripheral myelin. This segment of the nerve is 1–3 mm long, and it is also known as the Obersteiner–Redlich zone. The myelin sheath of the central nervous system portion is thinner than the peripheral portion, suggesting that the root exit zone is more susceptible to injury.

Extrinsic neural compression by a vascular loop promotes segmental demyelination, causing an ectopic synapse to occur—ephaptic or "cross-talk" transmission (Gardner 1966, Nielsen 1984). Moller (1991) showed that the entire central nervous system segment, including the nucleus, is triggered by an offending vascular loop, increasing discharge activity of the nerve. Surgical vascular decompression using insulating Teflon suppresses all vascular impacts to the hyperactive facial nerve.

**Diagnostic evaluation.** There is still controversy concerning the etiology, due to an inability in some cases to identify an offending vessel in spite of the illumination and magnification provided by the operating microscope. In addition, a vascular loop lying in contact with the acousticofacial nerve bundle is a common anatomical finding.

The supplementary information provided by cerebellopontine angle endoscopy is critically important to demonstrate the dynamics of the relationships between the acousticofacial nerve bundle and the adjacent vessels; to recognize the real offending vessel accurately; to detect multiple sites of vascular nerve compression; and to carry out vascular decompression safely and reliably (Fig. **71**).

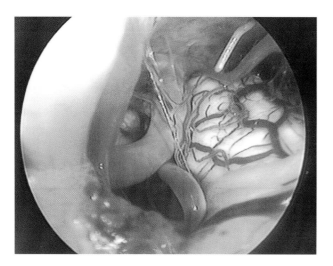 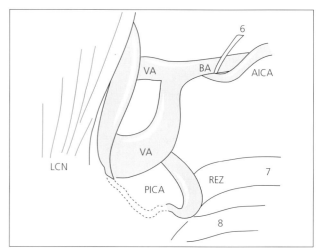

Fig. **71a, b**   The patient had been suffering from left hemifacial spasm for 14 years. The image shows that the root exit zone (REZ) of the facial nerve (7) is being stretched by the offending posterior inferior cerebellar artery. The vertebral artery is also involved in the vascular compression. Both the posterior inferior cerebellar artery and the vertebral artery have to be mobilized and positioned away from the REZ.

| | |
|---|---|
| 6 | Abducent nerve |
| 7 | Facial nerve |
| 8 | Vestibulocochlear nerve |
| AICA | Anterior inferior cerebellar artery |
| LCN | Lower cranial nerves |
| PICA | Posterior inferior cerebellar artery |
| REZ | Root entry zone |
| BA | Basilar artery |
| VA | Vertebral artery |

T1 and T2 three-dimensional Fourier transform (FT) MRI is the most effective method of delineating both the acousticofacial nerve bundle and the surrounding vascular structures in the cerebellopontine angle and the internal auditory canal. T2 is carried out using a with constructive interference in steady state (CISS) sequence (Fig. **72**).

The correlation between the imaging data and the operative findings was analyzed in the first 81 patients with hemifacial spasm whom we treated. In the 81 patients, neurovascular contact was identified by MRI in 76 cases (94%). The offending vessel caused stretching and deformity of neural structures in 35 of these 76 cases (46%)—in the facial nerve alone in 12 cases; in

the lateral part of the pons in six cases; and in both the pons and the nerve in 17 cases. Neurovascular contact without deformity was found in 41 of the 76 cases (54%)—at the root exit zone in 39 cases, and at the porus acusticus in two cases. Vascular compression was not identified in five cases. Surgery was carried out in all 81 patients, confirming vascular compression in 78 and a lack of neurovascular contact in three. MRI thus had a sensitivity of 97% and a specificity of 100%; the positive predictive value was 100%, and the negative predictive value was 60%. MRI is thus highly sensitive for depicting vascular compression of the facial nerve, and is a potentially important method of assessing the indication for surgical treatment.

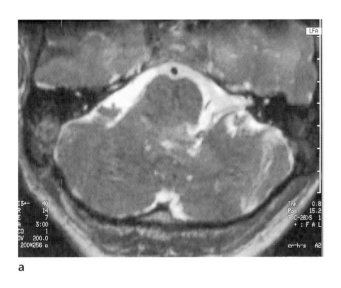

a

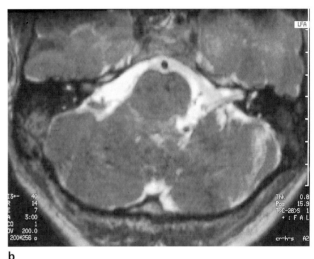

b

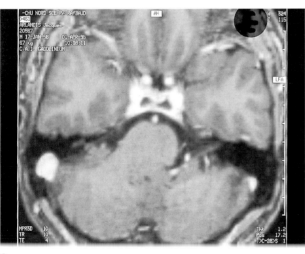

c

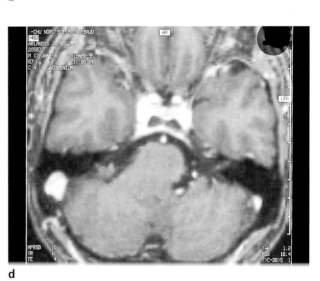

d

Fig. **72a–d**  Left hemifacial spasm. **a**, **b** Reformatted constructive interference in steady state (CISS) image in the axial plane. **c**, **d** Post-contrast reformatted turboflash in the axial plane. The compression is caused by the left vertebral artery, leading to deformities in both the pons and the root exit zone of the facial nerve.

## First Case: Vertebral Artery and Posterior Inferior Cerebellar Artery as Offending Vessels
(Figs. **73–79**)

This first case provides a summary of the various steps involved in the endoscopic procedure during retrosigmoid vascular decompression.

A 66-year-old man had been suffering from left hemifacial spasm for 11 years, and the condition had not responded to medical treatment. Botulinum toxin had been used for five years without benefit. MRI demonstrated that the vertebral artery and posterior inferior cerebellar artery were compressing the root exit zone of the facial nerve and the lateral bulbar fossa.

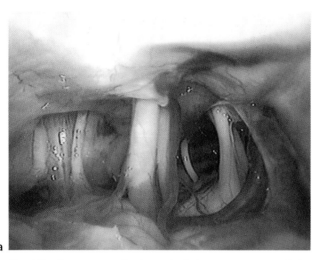

a

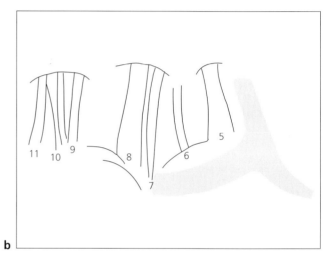

b

Fig. **73a, b**   Panoramic view of all the components of the cerebellopontine angle, with no modification of the neurovascular relationships.

5   Trigeminal nerve
6   Abducent nerve
7   Facial nerve
8   Vestibulocochlear nerve
9   Glossopharyngeal nerve
10   Vagus nerve
11   Accessory nerve

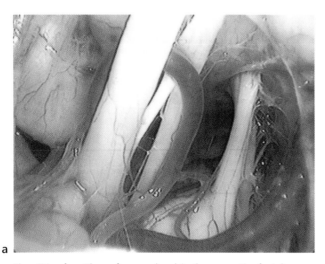

a

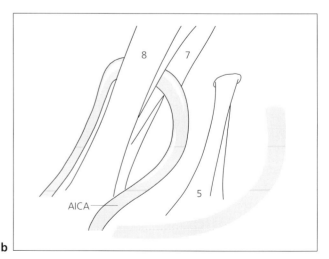

b

Fig. **74a, b**   The reference level is the acousticofacial nerve bundle. The anterior inferior cerebellar artery, lying between the auditory and facial nerves, is found in 38% of cases.

5      Trigeminal nerve
7      Facial nerve
8      Vestibulocochlear nerve
AICA   Anterior inferior cerebellar artery

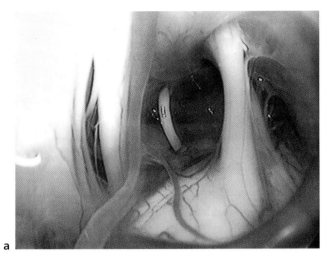

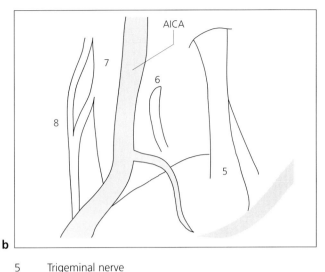

Fig. **75a, b**  The root of the facial nerve is exposed above the acousticofacial nerve bundle. In the background lies the trigeminal area.

| | |
|---|---|
| 5 | Trigeminal nerve |
| 6 | Abducent nerve |
| 7 | Facial nerve |
| 8 | Vestibulocochlear nerve |
| AICA | Anterior inferior cerebellar artery |

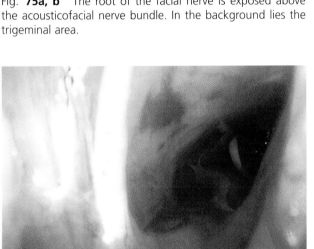

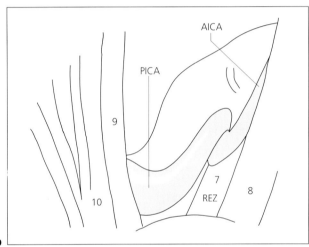

Fig. **76a, b**  Below the acousticofacial nerve bundle and above the lower cranial nerves, the root exit zone of the facial nerve is visualized, and the offending vessel (the posterior inferior cerebellar artery) is identified.

| | |
|---|---|
| 7 | Facial nerve |
| 8 | Vestibulocochlear nerve |
| 9 | Glossopharyngeal nerve |
| 10 | Vagus nerve |
| AICA | Anterior inferior cerebellar artery |
| PICA | Posterior inferior cerebellar artery |
| REZ | Root exit zone |

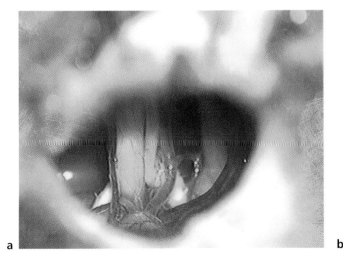

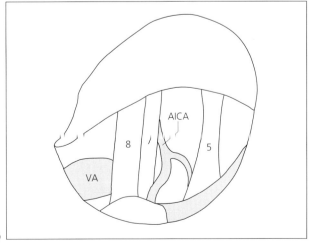

Fig. **77a, b**  Compare the view through the retrosigmoid craniotomy using the operating microscope (original magnification x 10).

| | |
|---|---|
| 5 | Trigeminal nerve |
| 7 | Facial nerve |
| 8 | Vestibulocochlear nerve |
| AICA | Anterior inferior cerebellar artery |
| VA | Vertebral artery |

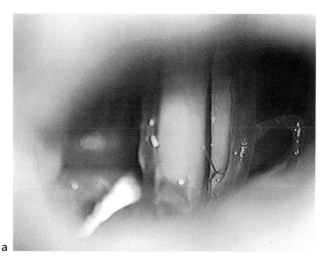

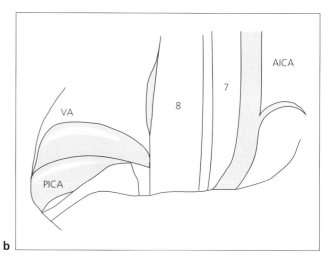

Fig. **78a, b**    Vascular decompression is carried out under the operating microscope.

7      Facial nerve
8      Vestibulocochlear nerve
AICA   Anterior inferior cerebellar artery
PICA   Posterior inferior cerebellar artery
VA     Vertebral artery

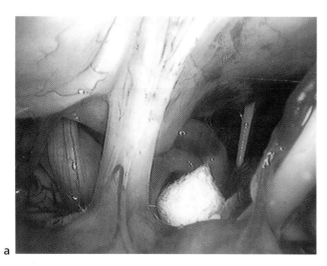

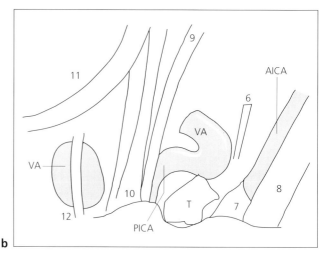

Fig. **79a, b**    Using the endoscope, the position of the Teflon pad and the efficacy of the vascular decompression is checked.

6      Abducent nerve
7      Facial nerve
8      Vestibulocochlear nerve
9      Glossopharyngeal nerve
10     Vagus nerve
11     Accessory nerve
12     Hypoglossal nerve
AICA   Anterior inferior cerebellar artery
PICA   Posterior inferior cerebellar artery
T      Teflon
VA     Vertebral artery

## Second Case: the Vertebral Artery as the Offending Vessel (Figs. 80–87)

A 63-year-old man had been suffering from left hemifacial spasm for eight years. MRI showed that the vertebral artery was compressing the root exit zone of the facial nerve. This case illustrates why neurovascular compression as a cause of hemifacial spasm can be overlooked even when the operating microscope is being used.

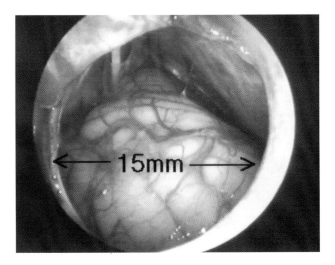

Fig. **80**  The craniotomy was a 15-mm circular trephination behind and close to the sigmoid sinus. The dura has been opened. The cerebellum has retracted spontaneously due to the effect of profound balanced anesthesia, with assisted hyperventilation.

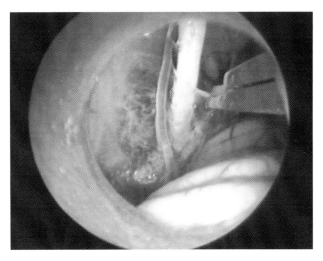

Fig. **81**  The arachnoid surrounding the acousticofacial nerve bundle is opened. The cerebrospinal fluid escapes from the basal cisterns and the cerebellum falls away without any pressure on it.

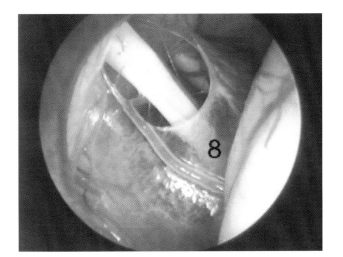

Fig. **82**  No vascular loop is visualized directly ahead.

8  Vestibulocochlear nerve

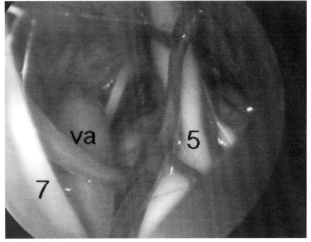

Fig. **83**  The tip of the endoscope is above the acousticofacial nerve bundle, allowing easy identification of the offending vessel (the vertebral artery) without the risks associated with retraction.

5   Trigeminal nerve
7   Facial nerve
va  Vertebral artery

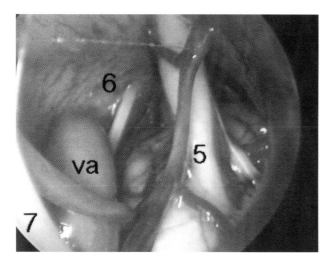

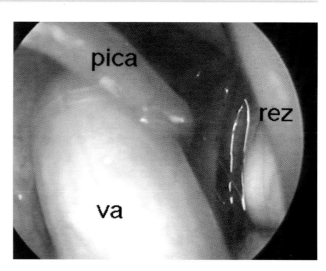

Fig. **84** Panoramic view of the trigeminal area. The vertebral artery is clearly compressing the root exit zone of the facial nerve in an inferior to superior direction.

5   Trigeminal nerve
6   Abducent nerve
7   Facial nerve
va  Vertebral artery

Fig. **85** Endoscopic view of the compression, below the acousticofacial nerve bundle. As it crosses, the vertebral artery is compressing the root exit zone of the facial nerve at right angles.

pica Posterior inferior cerebellar artery
rez  Root exit zone
va   Vertebral artery

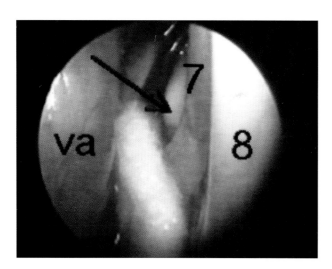

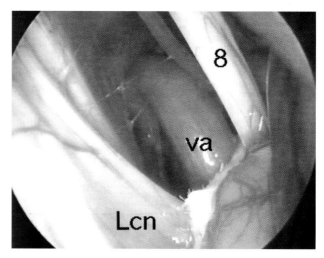

Fig. **86** Using an endoscope with a diameter of 2.7 mm and a 30° angled view, morphological changes are visualized in the neural appearance of the root of the facial nerve (arrow).

7   Facial nerve
8   Vestibulocochlear nerve
va  Vertebral artery

Fig. **87** The offending vertebral artery is held away from the root exit zone of the facial nerve using small Teflon foam pads, as recommended by Jannetta (1988).

8    Vestibulocochlear nerve
Lcn  Lower cranial nerves
va   Vertebral artery

## Third Case: a Dolichovertebral Artery as an Offending Vessel (Figs. 88–97)

A 37-year-old man had been suffering from facial spasm for three years. MRI demonstrated vascular compression by the vertebral artery, leading to deformities in both the lateral bulbar fossa and the root exit zone of the facial nerve.

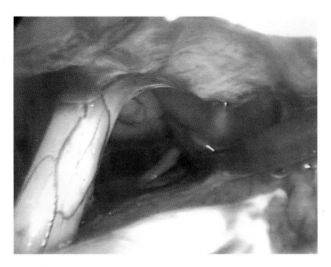

Fig. **88**  Endoscope 0°, diameter 4 mm, length 6 cm. The endoscope is inserted between the posterior wall of the petrous bone and the cerebellum. The acousticofacial nerve bundle is the endoscopic landmark; the offending vessels are seen underneath it.

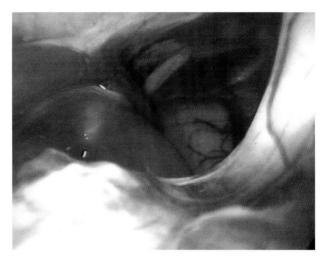

Fig. **89**  Below the acousticofacial nerve, the vertebral artery is partly hidden by the flocculonodular lobe and embedded in the neural structure.

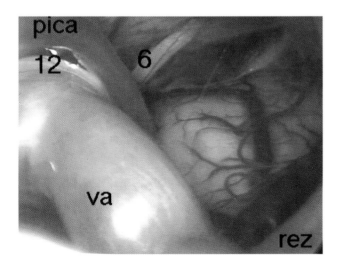

Fig. **90**  The root exit zone of the facial nerve and the vascular loop of the vertebral artery are visualized.

 6  Abducent nerve
12  Hypoglossal nerve
rez  Root exit zone
va  Vertebral artery

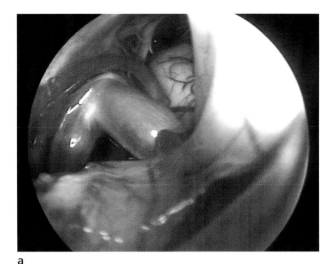

a

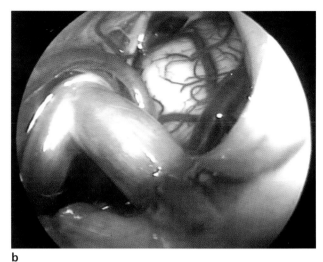

b

Fig. **91a–c**  Endoscopic angled view 30°, diameter 4 mm. The angle of view onto the root exit zone of the acoustico-facial nerve bundle is better, and provides a better assessment of the vascular structures affecting the facial nerve.

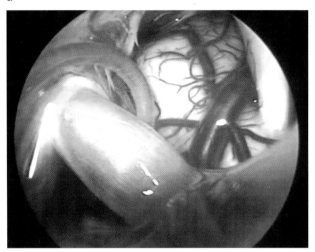

c

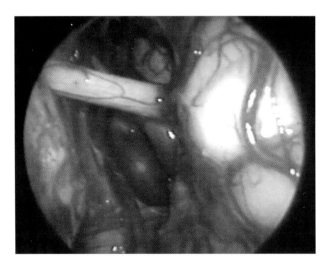

Fig. **92**  Endoscopic view, 30° optical system, diameter 2.7 mm. Reducing the diameter of the endoscope allows better maneuverability in the cerebellopontine angle, without touching the neural structures. Shown here is an overview of the cerebellopontine angle. At the top lies the trigeminal nerve; in the middle, the acousticofacial nerve bundle; under it are the left and right vertebral arteries; at the bottom lies the lower cranial nerves.

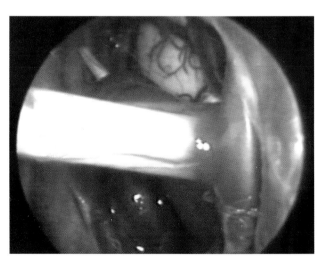

Fig. **93**  The endoscope is facing the auditory nerve. Above it lies the trigeminal area, and below it the lower cranial nerve area.

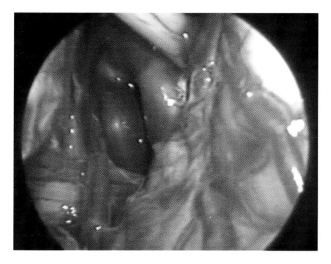

Fig. **94**  The lower cranial nerves, both vertebral arteries, and the posterior inferior cerebellar artery are well exposed.

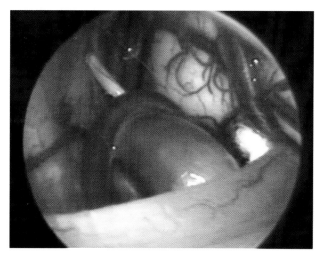

Fig. **95**  Endoscopic checking of vascular decompression using an angled-view 30° endoscope, diameter 2.8 mm. The angled-view 30° endoscope allows inspection of the superior aspect of the facial nerve. Correct positioning of the Teflon pad can be checked from above.

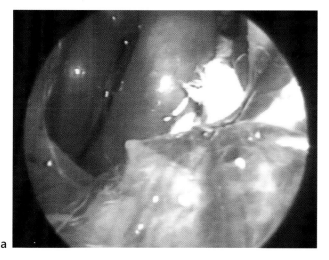

a

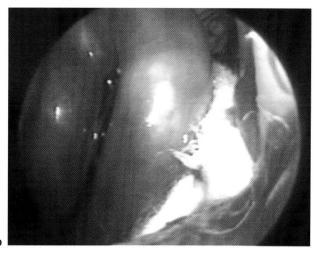

b

Fig. **96a, b**  The angled-view 30° endoscope, viewing from behind, allows the efficacy of the vascular decompression between the vertebral artery and the root exit zone to be confirmed. The tip of the endoscope can be used to mobilize the

offending vessel carefully in order to check the exact location of the Teflon pad insulating the facial nerve in the vicinity of the vascular loops.

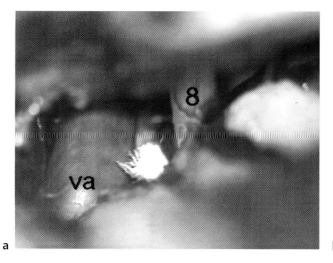

a

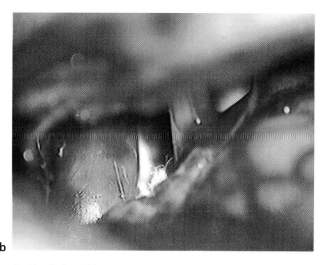

b

Fig. **97a, b**  Surgical views, for comparison with the above endoscopic assessments.

8   Vestibulocochlear nerve
va  Vertebral artery

## Fourth Case: the Posterior Inferior Cerebellar Artery as the Offending Vessel (Figs. 98–105)

A 62-year-old woman had been suffering from left hemifacial spasm for six years. Botulinum toxin treatment had been tried for two years. MRI demonstrated an obvious neurovascular compression by the posterior inferior cerebellar artery, causing a deformity in the root exit zone of the facial nerve.

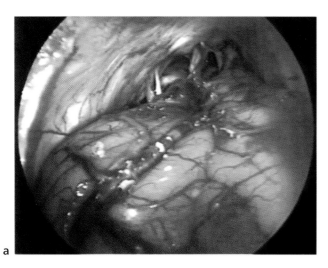

a

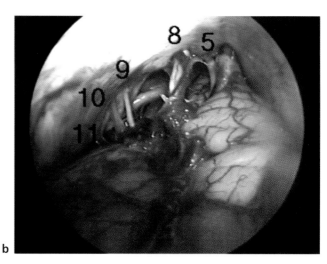

b

Fig. **98a, b**  Endoscopic overview of the left cerebellopontine angle with an angled-view 30° optical system, diameter 4 mm. The neurovascular bundles of the trigeminal (5), acousticofacial (8), and lower cranial nerves (9, 10, 11), are identified. In the background lie the offending vascular structures.

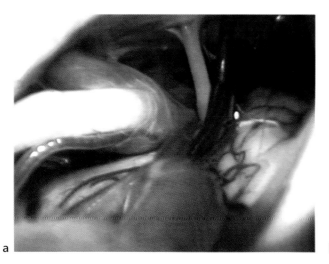

a

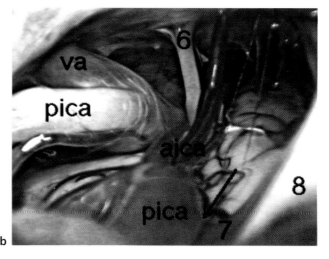

b

Fig. **99a, b**  The tip of a straight-viewing endoscope is positioned between the acousticofacial bundle and the lower cranial nerves. The offending vessel stretching the root exit zone of the facial nerve (arrow) is a loop of the posterior inferior cerebellar artery, which arises from the vertebral artery.
**a** Normal video, **b** Digivideo.

6    Abducent nerve
7    Facial nerve
8    Vestibulocochlear nerve
aica  Anterior inferior cerebellar artery
pica  Posterior inferior cerebellar artery
va    Vertebral artery

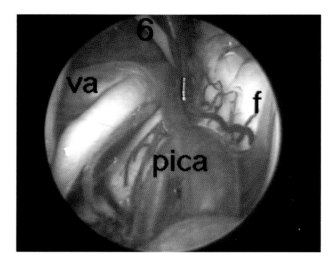

Fig. **100** Using an angled-view 30°endoscope, diameter 2.7 mm, provides accurate visualization of the neurovascular relationships.

6       Abducent nerve
f       Facial nerve
pica   Posterior inferior cerebellar artery
va     Vertebral artery

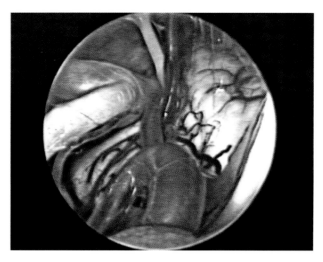

Fig. **101** The same view using Digivideo.

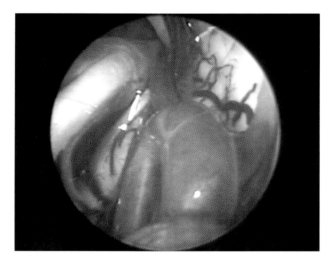

Fig. **102** The vascular loop of the posterior inferior cerebellar artery is concealing the root exit zone of the facial nerve and the anterior inferior cerebellar artery.

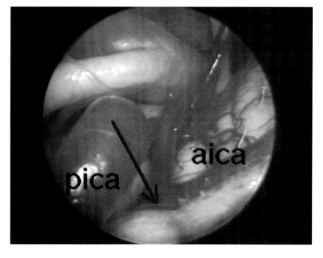

Fig. **103** After the posterior inferior cerebellar artery has been mobilized, the course of the anterior inferior cerebellar artery, in contact (arrow) with the root exit zone of the facial nerve, is identified on the endoscopic view.

aica   Anterior inferior cerebellar artery
pica   Posterior inferior cerebellar artery

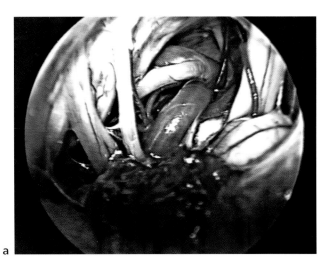
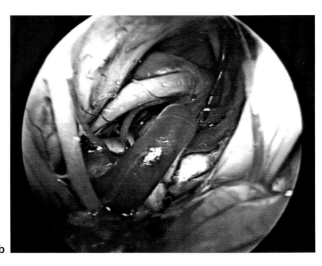

Fig. **104a, b**   Endoscopic checking of vascular decompression of both the posterior inferior and anterior inferior cerebellar arteries. All vessels that are in contact with the facial nerve have to be elevated and held away from the nerve to prevent renewed contact.

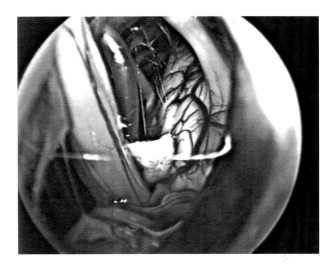

Fig. **105**   Withdrawing the endoscope. The efficacy of the vascular decompression is again confirmed from above the acousticofacial nerve bundle. The Teflon pad inserted between the facial nerve and the anterior inferior cerebellar artery is clearly seen, isolating the nerve from the pathological vessels.

## Fifth Case: Multiple Offending Vessels
(Figs. **106–108**)

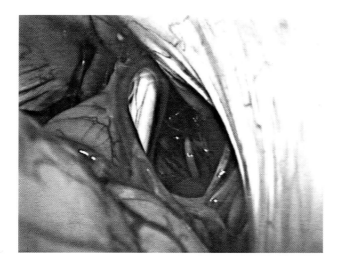

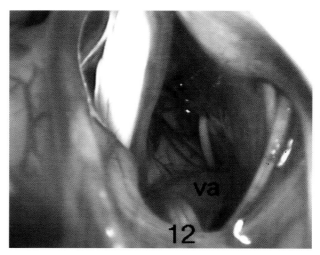

Fig. **106a, b** Endoscopic view of the right cerebellopontine angle between the acousticofacial nerve bundle and the lower cranial nerves. The vertebral artery is seen displacing the hypoglossal nerve (endoscope 0°, diameter 4 mm).

12 Hypoglossal nerve
va Vertebral artery

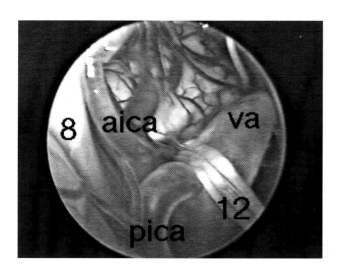

Fig. **107** Using an angled-view 30° endoscope, diameter 2.8 mm, multiple offending vessels are seen stretching the root exit zone of the facial nerve.

8 Vestibulocochlear nerve
12 Hypoglossal nerve
aica Anterior inferior cerebellar artery
pica Posterior inferior cerebellar artery
va Vertebral artery

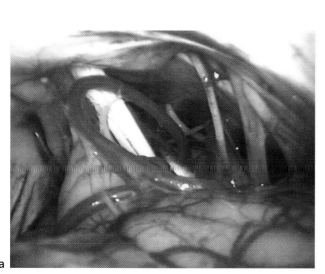

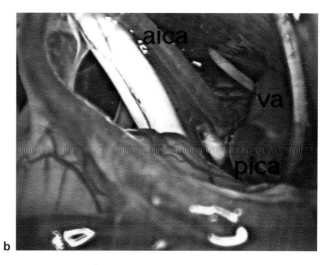

a

b

Fig. **108a, b** Endoscopic control after microvascular decompression of the offending vessels. The same view using normal video (**a**) and Digivideo (**b**).

aica Anterior inferior cerebellar artery
pica Posterior inferior cerebellar artery
va Vertebral artery

## Sixth Case: Posterior Inferior Cerebellar Artery and Vertebral Artery as Offending Vessels
(Figs. **109–116**)

In a 57-year-old woman who had been suffering left hemifacial spasm for two years, MRI demonstrated an obvious neurovascular compression.

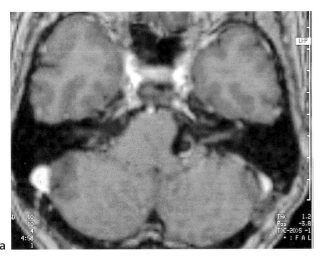

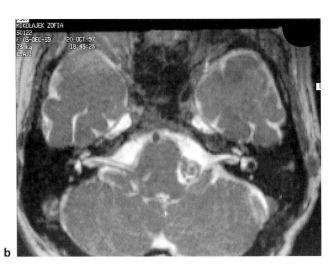

Fig. **109a, b** The T1 turboflash (**a**) and T2 CISS (**b**) sequences show the posterior inferior cerebellar artery and the vertebral artery causing distortion of both the lateral bul- bar fossa and the medial part of the acousticofacial nerve bundle.

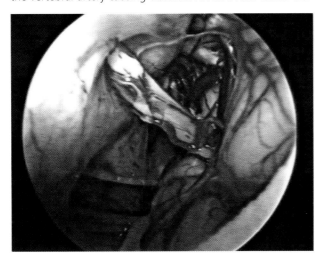

Fig. **110** Endoscopic view of the left cerebellopontine angle; no offending vessels are evident.

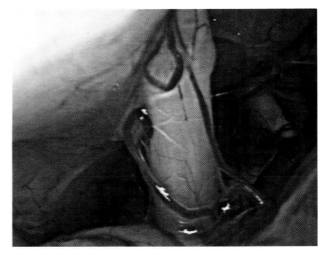

Fig. **111** Closer view of the acousticofacial nerve bundle.

Fig. **112** Using a 30° angled endoscope, the compression site (arrow) is identified above the acousticofacial nerve bundle.

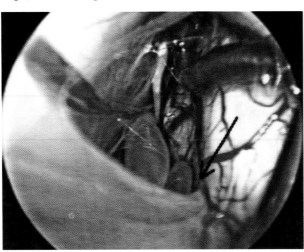

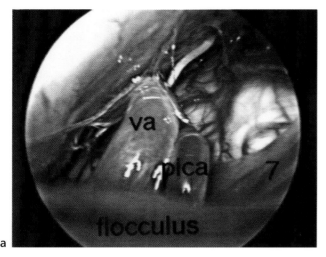
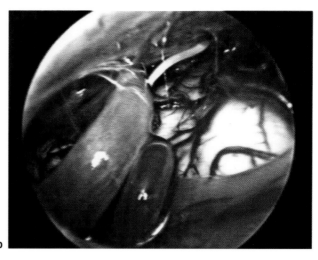

a

b

Fig. **113a, b** The endoscope is positioned below the acousticofacial nerve bundle. The root exit zone of the facial nerve is being compressed by both the posterior inferior cerebellar artery and the vertebral artery.

7     Facial nerve
pica  Posterior inferior cerebellar artery
va    Vertebral artery

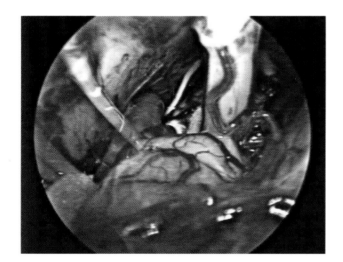
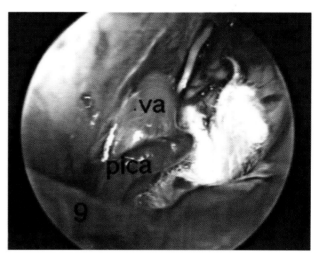

Fig. **114**   Endoscopic checking after microvascular decompression.

Fig. **115**   Compare this view with Fig. **113**.

9     Glossopharyngeal nerve
pica  Posterior inferior cerebellar artery
va    Vertebral artery

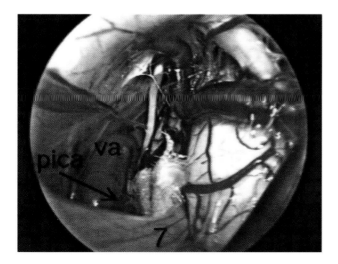

Fig. **116**   Compare this view with Fig. **112**.

7     Facial nerve
pica  Posterior inferior cerebellar artery
va    Vertebral artery

## Seventh Case: the Anterior Inferior Cerebellar Artery as the Offending Vessel (Figs. 117–119)

Our intraoperative endoscopic criteria for cross-conflicts are as follows:

1   Site of the lesion. The vascular loop cross-compresses the root exit zone of the facial nerve at right angles, causing distortion of the root zone and/or distortion of the neural structure of the lateral bulbar fossa and inferior lip of the pons.
2   Dynamic action. The offending vessels usually stretch the nerve from a caudal to a rostral direction.

3   Neural appearance. There are morphological changes in the color and appearance of the root of the facial nerve.

In 124 cases of hemifacial spasm, it was possible to identify 121 vascular compressions using these endoscopic criteria. The precise location of the offending vessel was apparent using the operating microscope alone in only 28% of these cases. The endoscopic procedure thus provided an additional 72% accuracy rate for the diagnosis, without dislocation of the acoustico-facial nerve bundle and retraction of the cerebellum.

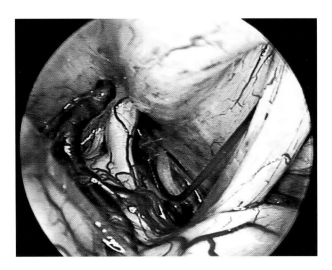

Fig. **117**   The initial inspection of the cerebellopontine angle did not reveal an obvious offending vessel.

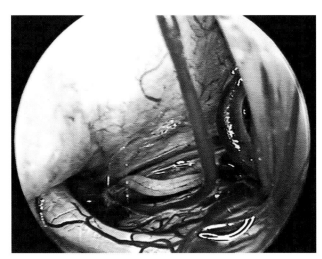

Fig. **118**   The tip of the endoscope is positioned close to and above the acousticofacial nerve bundle, allowing visualization of the loop of the anterior inferior cerebellar artery, which is compressing the root of the facial nerve.

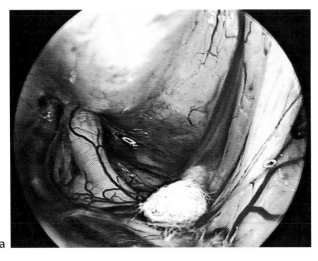

a

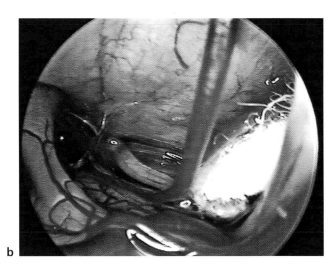

b

Fig. **119a, b**   Endoscopic inspection after microvascular decompression. The Teflon pad is holding the anterior inferi-or cerebellar artery away, isolating the nerve from all vascular structures.

## References

Fukushima T. Vascular decompression syndromes. Paper presented at the Second International Skull Base Congress, North American Skull Base Society, San Diego, California, 29 June–4 July 1996.

Gardner W. Five-year cure of hemifacial spasm. Cleve Clin Q 1960; 27: 219–21.

Gardner WJ. Cross talk: the paradoxical transmission of a nerve impulse. Arch Neurol 1966; 14: 149–56.

Girard N, Poncet M, Chays A, Tallon Y, Raybaud C, Magnan J. Neurovascular compression in the CP angle. Riv Neuroradiol 1995; 8: 981–9.

Jannetta P. The cause of hemifacial spasm: definitive microsurgical treatment at the brainstem in 31 patients. Trans Am Acad Ophthalmol Otol 1975; 80: 319–22.

Jannetta P. Neurovascular contact in hemifacial spasm. In: Portmann M, ed. Facial nerve. Paris: Masson, 1985: 45–8.

Jannetta P. Microvascular decompression for hemifacial spasm. In: May M, ed. The facial nerve. New York: Thieme, 1988: 499–508.

Magnan J, Chays A, Caces F. Place de l'endoscopie et de la décompression vasculaire dans le traitement du spasme de l'hémiface. Ann Otolaryngol (Paris) 1994; 111: 153–60.

Magnan J, Chays A, Caces F, Locatelli P. Hemifacial spasm: endoscopic vascular decompression. In: Sterkers JM, Sterkers O, Charachon R, eds. Proceedings of the Second International Conference on Acoustic Neuroma and Second European Skull Base Society Congress, Paris. Amsterdam: Kugler, 1996: 439–44.

Magnan J, Caces F, Locatelli P, Chays A. Hemifacial spasm: endoscopic vascular decompression. Otolaryngol Head Neck Surg 1997; 117: 308–14.

Moller AR. Interaction between the blink reflex and the abnormal muscle response in patients with hemifacial spasm: results of intraoperative recordings. J Neurol Sci 1991; 101: 114–23.

Nielsen V. Pathophysiology of hemifacial spasm. Neurology 1984; 34: 418–31.

Raybaud C, Girard N, Poncet M, Chays A, Caces F, Magnan J. L'imagerie actuelle des conflits vasculo-nerveux de l'angle pontocérébelleux. Rev Laryngol Otol Rhinol 1995; 116: 99–103.

Schwaber M. Vascular compression syndrome. In: Jackler R, Brackmann D, eds. Neuro-otology. St Louis: Mosby, 1993: 881–903.

Wilkins R. Hemifacial spasm: a review. Surg Neurol 1991; 36: 251–77.

Zhang KW, Shun ZT. Microvascular decompression by the retrosigmoid approach for idiopathic hemifacial spasm: experience with 300 cases. Ann Otol Rhinol Laryngol 1995; 104: 106–12.

## Trigeminal Neuralgia

Trigeminal neuralgia, or "tic douloureux," is characterized by severe and intense facial pain triggered by tactile stimulation of the face. Vascular compression in the cerebellopontine angle, as in the case of hemifacial spasm, was first proposed by Dandy (1984) as an explanation of the pathogenesis of trigeminal neuralgia. Compression of the root entry zone by a vascular loop (Fig. **120**) results in demyelination and deactivation of the inhibitory fibers of the trigeminal nerve. Tactile stimuli on the face then cause hyperactivity of the trigeminal nucleus, and subsequent increased discharge of the trigeminal nerve results in intense pain.

**Diagnostic evaluation.** Dandy described the superior cerebellar artery as affecting the nerve in 30% of his 215 cases of trigeminal neuralgia. The introduction of the operating microscope was a major advance, allowing arterial compression of the trigeminal nerve and root entry zone to be identified in 80% of patients. A vein alone was responsible for trigeminal neuralgia in 10% of cases. The endoscope provides a panoramic view of the entire course of the nerve, from the pons to the Meckel cavity. The Meckel cavity, the root entry zone, and the proximal segment of the artery loop all have to be inspected without disturbing the neurovascular relationships.

Neurovascular contact, corresponding to the extent of the trigeminal neuralgia, was identified using MRI in 25 of 35 patients. The offending vessel was the superior cerebellar artery in 17 patients and veins in six, without any deformity in the trigeminal nerve itself. In the two remaining cases, a distended basilar artery was the cause of the deformity in the fifth nerve. The cross-conflict was at the root exit zone in nine cases, at the cisternal course of the nerve in 12, and at the Meckel cavity in four. Identification of the offending vessel was confirmed by surgery in all cases, and both the superior cerebellar artery and veins were found to be responsible in three cases.

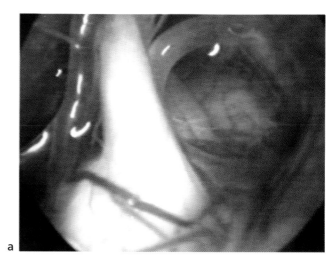

a

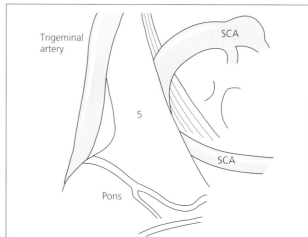

b

Fig. **120a, b**   Endoscope 0°, diameter 4 mm, length 6 cm, used through a left keyhole retrosigmoid approach for a patient suffering from left trigeminal neuralgia. A loop of the trunk of the superior cerebellar artery is seen deforming the superomedial side of the trigeminal nerve at the root entry zone.

5    Trigeminal nerve
SCA  Superior cerebellar artery

## First Case (Figs. **121–124**)

This case summarizes the different steps of the endoscopic procedure and indicates the key aspects of vascular decompression in a patient with right trigeminal neuralgia.

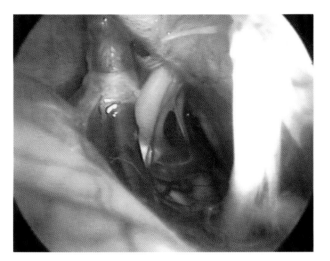

Fig. **121**  Exposure of the trigeminal area. The vascular compression is evaluated endoscopically, without disturbing the neurovascular relationships.

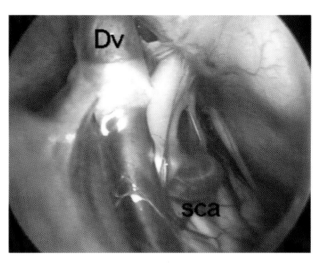

Fig. **122**  Identification of the offending vessel. The superior petrosal vein or the Dandy vein (Dv) is in the surgeon's way, but is not touching the nerve. The superior cerebellar artery (sca) is the offending vessel at the root entry zone of the trigeminal nerve.

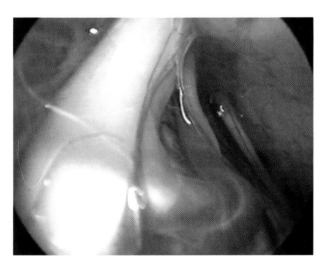

Fig. **123**  Exposure of the neurovascular cross-conflict. The trigeminal nerve is being compressed by a loop of the superior cerebellar artery dangling down into the axilla of the nerve and distorting it.

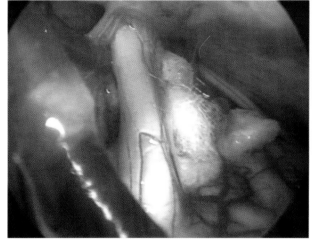

Fig. **124**  Decompression surgery. The offending vessel is moved away from the trigeminal nerve, and the separation is maintained using a small Teflon pad to protect the nerve's medial and superior surfaces.

## Second Case: Superior Cerebellar Artery as the Offending Vessel (Figs. 125–132)

A 70-year-old woman had been suffering from left trigeminal neuralgia for three years, and medical treatment had failed. MRI demonstrated that the superior cerebellar artery was compressing the trigeminal nerve root.

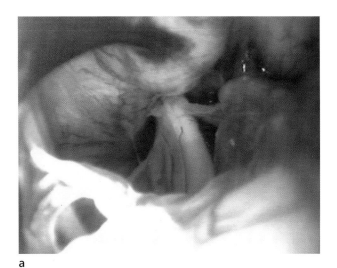

a

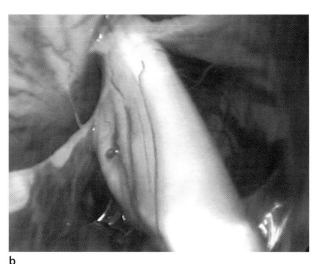

b

Fig. **125a–c** Endoscope 0°, diameter 4 mm, length 6 cm. The offending vessel is the superior cerebellar artery, on the superomedial side of the trigeminal nerve. The nerve is deeply grooved and stretched by the arterial loop.

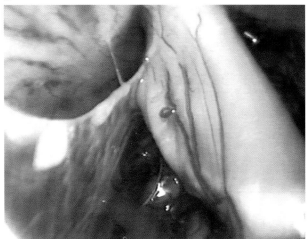

c

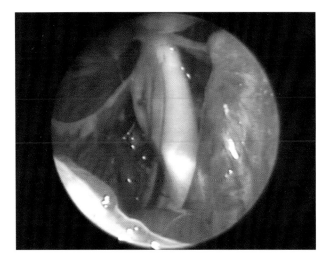

Fig. **126** Endoscope 30°, diameter 2.7 mm. Overview of the trigeminal area. The Dandy vein is adjacent to the trigeminal nerve and is not obstructing the view of an obvious vascular compression.

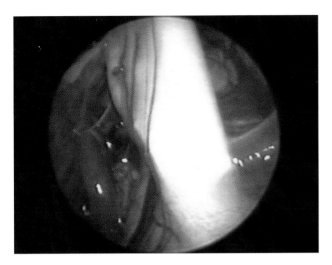

Fig. **127** The superior cerebellar artery has looped down into the axilla between the medial side and the pons. The course of the superior cerebellar artery is only visible from the surgeon's line of view at the root entry zone of the nerve.

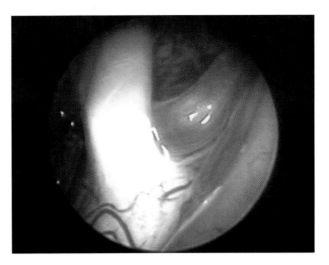

Fig. **128** The endoscope provides a view of the compression zone along the medial and superior surfaces of the nerve and the pons.

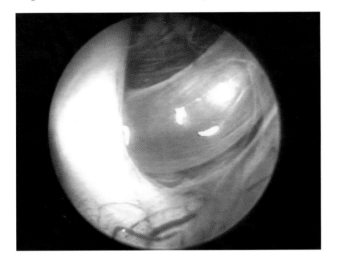

Fig. **129** Nerve angulation at the root entry zone of the trigeminal nerve.

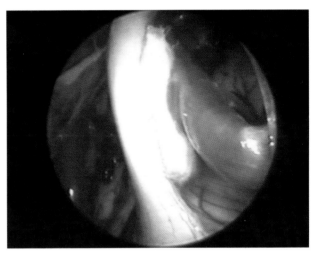

Fig. **130** The superior cerebellar artery is gently elevated away from the trigeminal nerve. Separation of the superior surface of the nerve and the artery is maintained using a small Teflon foam pad.

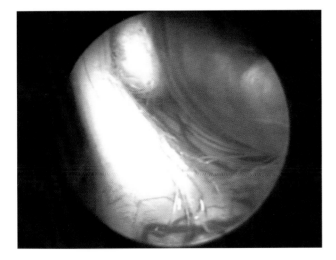

Fig. **131** An endoscopic check shows that the arterial loop is lying in a vertical position alongside the Teflon, and thus pressing on the nerve secondarily.

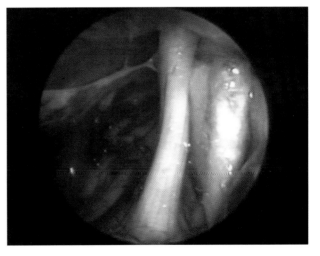

Fig. **132** The axis of the vascular loop is completely mobilized so that the superior cerebellar artery lies horizontally under the tentorium. In the resulting horizontal configuration, the outside of the loop is not pulsating against the nerve. The normal course of the trigeminal nerve has been restored.

## Third Case: Multiple Offending Vessels
(Figs. **133–139**)

A 64-year-old woman had been suffering from left trigeminal neuralgia for 11 years, and the condition had been refractory to medical treatment, radiofrequency thermal coagulation, and balloon compression.

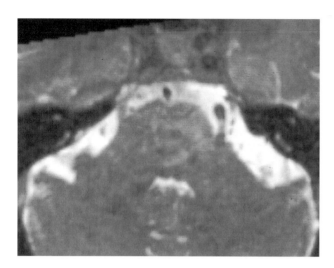

Fig. **133**   MR imaging demonstrated obvious neurovascular compression by a distended vertebral artery and a superior cerebellar artery, resulting in distortion of the trigeminal nerve.

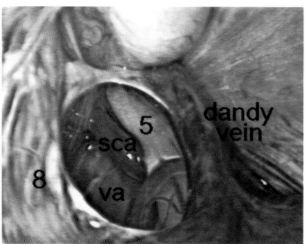

a

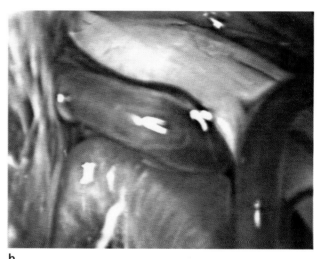

b

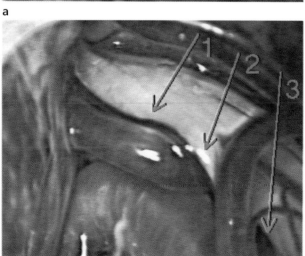

c

Fig. **134a–c**   Endoscopic views of the upper part of the cerebellopontine angle show an obvious deformity of the trigeminal nerve, which is being compressed from inferior to superior by the superior cerebellar artery and a tortuous vertebral artery, and from superior to inferior by a branch of the superior cerebellar artery. The multiple offending vessels are producing three compression sites—from the superior cerebellar artery (1); between the superior cerebellar artery and its branch (2); and from the vertebral artery (3).

5   Trigeminal nerve
8   Vestibulocochlear nerve
sca Superior cerebellar artery
va  Vertebral artery

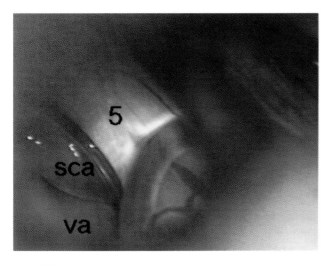

Fig. **135** The same view through the operating microscope, demonstrating the importance of a comprehensive evaluation of the entire nerve from the Meckel cavity to the pons. Here, the lateral and the medial segments of the trigeminal nerve are not visible from the surgeon s line of view.

5    Trigeminal nerve
sca  Superior cerebellar artery
va   Vertebral artery

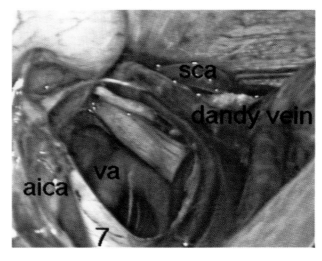

Fig. **136** The object of the surgical procedure was to change the axis of the superior cerebellar artery from inferior to superior, so that the superior cerebellar artery would lie horizontally under the tentorium. The Teflon pads are placed along the trigeminal nerve and Dandy vein.

7    Facial nerve
aica Anterior inferior cerebellar artery
sca  Superior cerebellar artery
va   Vertebral artery

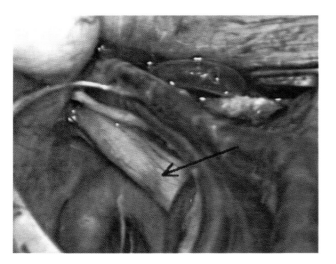

Fig. **137** Note the atrophic appearance (arrow) of the trigeminal nerve, due to the vascular compression.

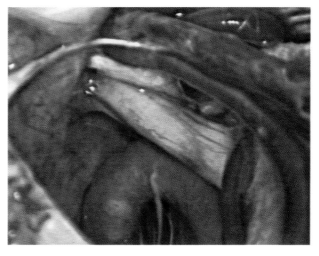

Fig. **138** The tortuous elongation of the vertebral artery is still impinging on the root entry of the trigeminal nerve, and requires specific decompression.

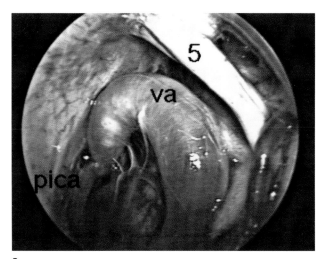

a

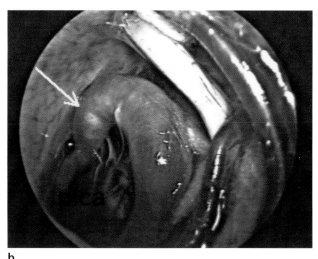

b

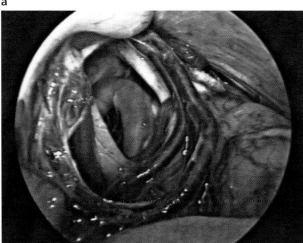

c

Fig. **139a–c**   The final endoscopic inspection using an angled-view 30° endoscope, diameter 4 mm. Note the arteriosclerotic appearance of the dolichovertebral artery (arrow in **b**). (**c**) View using a 0° endoscope.

5      Trigeminal nerve
pica   Posterior inferior cerebellar artery
va     Vertebral artery

## Fourth Case: Venous Compression (Figs. 140–143)

A 37-year-old woman had been suffering from left trigeminal neuralgia for six months, and medical treatment had failed.

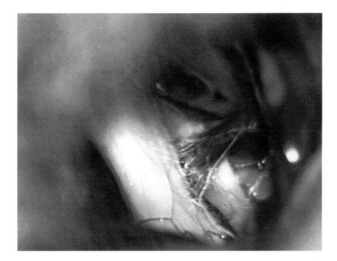

Fig. **140**   Left retrosigmoid approach. A vein is piercing the root of the trigeminal nerve, and then passing to the superior petrosal sinus adjacent to the Dandy vein.

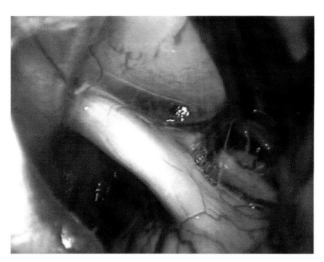

Fig. **141**   Endoscopic view of the trigeminal area, showing a trigeminal vein going through the root entry zone of the trigeminal nerve, without any other offending vessels.

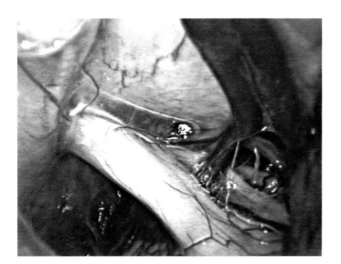

Fig. **142**   The same endoscopic view, using Digivideo.

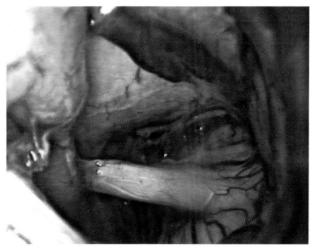

Fig. **143**   Coagulation and section of the offending vein. The normal course of the trigeminal nerve is restored. The trochlear nerve is visible in the background, adjacent to the tentorium.

## Fifth Case: Superior Cerebellar Artery and
## Trigeminal Vein (Figs. 144–145)

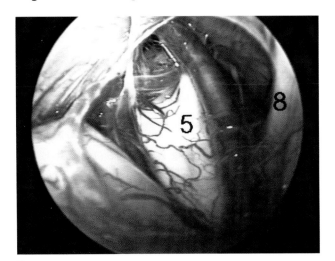

a

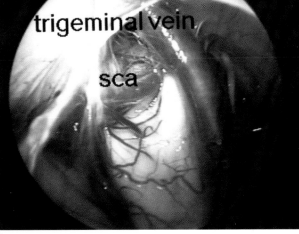

b

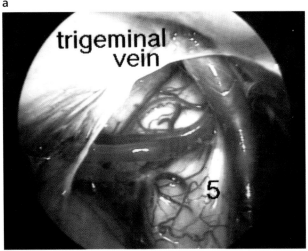

c

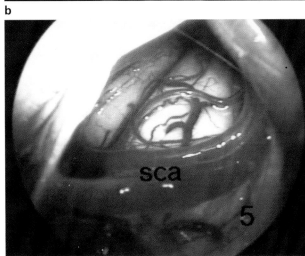

d

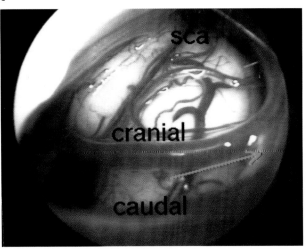

e

Fig. **144a–e** Progressive exploration of the trigeminal area, revealing a trigeminal vein and an offending superior cerebellar artery.

5   Trigeminal nerve
8   Vestibulocochlear nerve
sca   Superior cerebellar artery

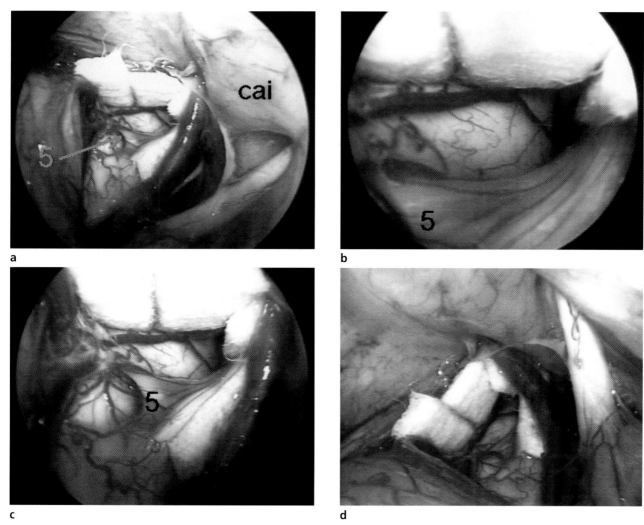

Fig. **145a–d** Endoscopic inspection after microvascular decompression of the trigeminal nerve, first using a 30° angled endoscope, and then a 0° endoscope.

5   Trigeminal nerve
cai  Internal auditory canal

## Sixth Case: Recurrent Pain after Surgical Treatment (Figs. 146–158)

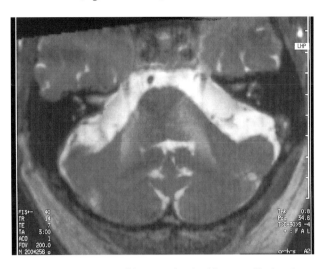

Fig. **146** A 79-year-old man who had been suffering from left trigeminal neuralgia for six years. In the reformatted CISS image in the axial plane, a vascular loop of the superior cerebellar artery is evident in the Meckel cavity and inferior to the trigeminal nerve.

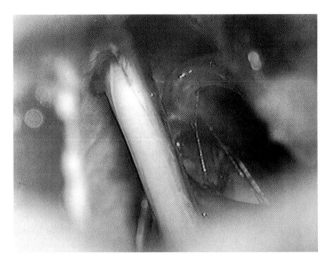

Fig. **147** Surgical findings under the operating microscope. There is a tortuous superior cerebellar artery compressing the trigeminal nerve anteriorly. It is difficult to identify the artery that is compressing the nerve.

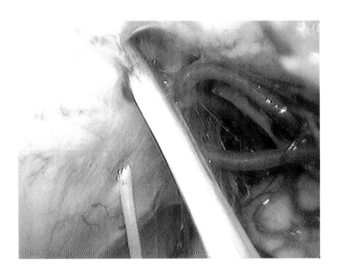

Fig. **148** In the endoscopic view, the distal nerve adjacent to the Meckel cavity is clearly visualized. There is a bifurcation of the superior cerebellar artery and its caudal trunk, causing compression of the trigeminal nerve.

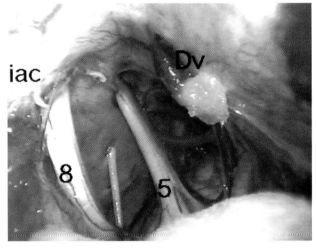

Fig. **149** Panoramic view of the trigeminal area; endoscope 0°, diameter 4 mm. The acousticofacial nerve bundle (8) is in the foreground. The Dandy vein was coagulated with gentle bipolar coagulation and sectioned near its junction with the superior petrosal sinus.

5    Trigeminal nerve
8    Vestibulocochlear nerve
Dv   Dandy vein
iac  Internal auditory canal

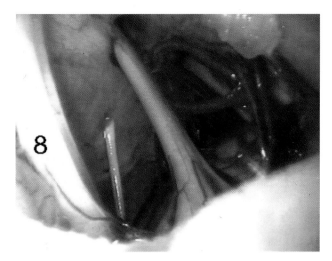

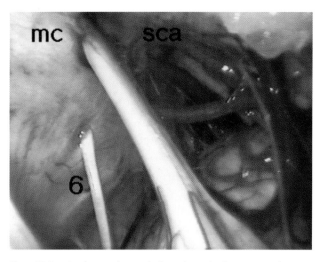

Fig. **150** The tip of the endoscope lies just above the acousticofacial nerve bundle (8). The site of the superior cerebellar artery compression of the trigeminal nerve is at the junction of the main trunk with the origin of the rostral and caudal trunks.

Fig. **151** A closer view of the trigeminal nerve and compression by the superior cerebellar artery adjacent to the Meckel cavity. Inferiorly, the abducent nerve is seen. The oculomotor nerve lies superiorly in the background.

6    Abducent nerve          sca  Superior cerebellar artery
mc  Meckel cavity

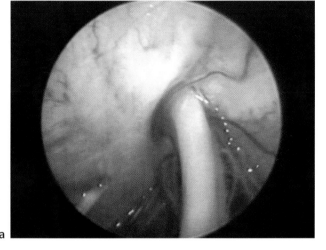

a

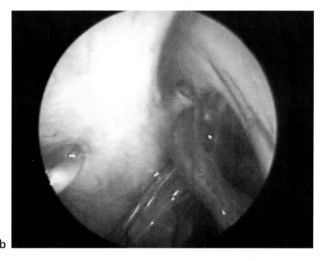

b

Fig. **152a, b**   Using an angled 30° endoscope, diameter 2.7 mm, the relationships between the distal part of the trigemi-

nal nerve adjacent to the Meckel cavity and the offending vessel are well visualized.

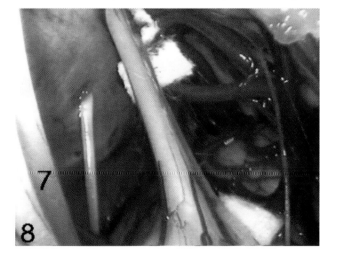

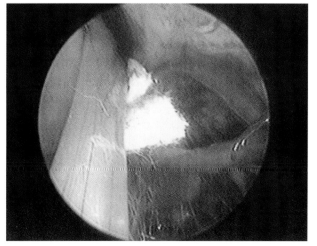

Fig. **153a, b**   All vessels making contact with, or in the vicinity of, the trigeminal nerve are carefully elevated from surface of the nerve. This requires division of arachnoidal adhesions under the operating microscope. Small Teflon pads are inserted between the nerve and the vessel to prevent renewed con-

tact. The effectiveness of the vascular decompression can be assessed using a straight-viewing 4-mm endoscope, and then a 30° angled view with a 2.7-mm endoscope.

7  Facial nerve                8  Vestibulocochlear nerve

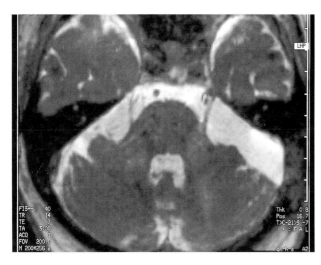

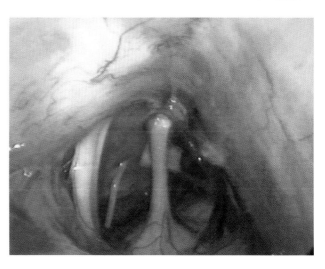

Fig. **154** Postoperative MRI. The reformatted CISS image in the axial plane provides a good demonstration of the vascular mobilization compared to the preoperative MRI, but a deformity of the nerve adjacent to the Meckel cavity still persists.

Fig. **155** Recurrence of pain made a second operative procedure necessary.

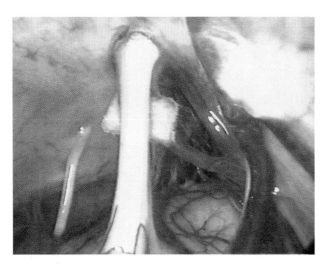

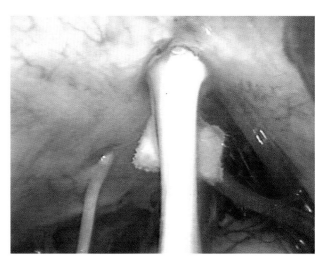

Fig. **156** The surgical findings during the repeated exploration. The arterial loop of the superior cerebellar artery has pushed one of the pieces of Teflon into the Meckel cavity, causing nerve angulation at the porus of the Meckel cavity, as the MRI suggested.

Fig. **157** Compare this view with the endoscopic view of the previous operation. The most anterior Teflon pad is not visible at all, and the trigeminal nerve is being compressed by the arterial loop in the Meckel cavity. Note the absence of adhesions and fibrous tissue surrounding the Teflon implant that was initially inserted.

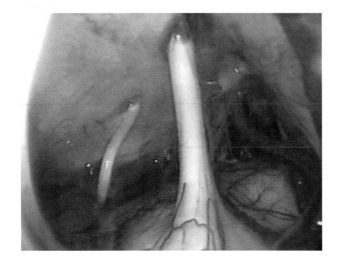

Fig. **158** The superior cerebellar loop and the Teflon material had adhered to trigeminal fascicles, which were sharply incised using microscissors. The arterial loop was mobilized slightly rostrally, from a vertical position to a horizontal one. The trigeminal nerve and the Meckel cavity are now free of compression.

# References

Apfelbaum RI. Surgery for tic douloureux. Clin Neurosurg 1983; 31: 351–68.

Dandy W. Concerning the cause of trigeminal neuralgia. Am J Surg 1984; 24: 447–55.

Fukushima T. Vascular compression syndromes. Paper presented at the Second International Skull Base Congress, North American Skull Base Society, San Diego, California, 29 June–4 July 1996.

Girard N, Poncet M, Chays A, Tallon Y, Raybaud C, Magnan J. Neurovascular compression in the CP angle. Riv Neuroradiol 1995; 8: 981–9.

Jannetta P. Microsurgery of cranial nerve cross-compression. Clin Neurosurg 1979; 26: 607–15.

Jannetta P. Neurovascular compression in cranial nerve and systemic disease. Ann Surg 1980; 192: 518–25.

Magnan J, Chays A, Cohen OM, Caces F, Locatelli P. Endoscopy of the cerebellopontine angle. Am J Otol 1995; 116: 115–8.

Rovit R, Murali R, Jannetta P. Trigeminal neuralgia. Baltimore: Williams and Wilkins, 1990.

Schwaber M. Vascular compression syndromes. In: Jackler A, Brackmann D, eds. Neuro-otology. St. Louis: Mosby, 1993: 881–903.

Sindou M, Keravel Y, Abdennebi B, Szapiro J. Traitement neuro-chirurgical de la névralgie trigeminale. Abord direct ou méthode percutanée. Neurochirurgie 1987; 33: 89–111.

Zhang KW, Zhao YH, Shun ZT, Li P. Microvascular decompression by retrosigmoid approach for trigeminal neuralgia: experience in 200 patients. Ann Otol Rhinol Laryngol 1990; 99: 129–30.

# ▩ Acoustic Neuroma

As House, Gardner, and Hughes stated in 1968, "The major principle of acoustic neuroma surgery is removal of the tumor without producing additional neurological damage." This principle provides the basis for the preservation of hearing. Hearing preservation became possible as a result of improvements in imaging techniques, allowing tumors to be detected when they are still small. Advances in the intraoperative management of acoustic neuromas have also greatly reduced the incidence of postoperative neurological deficits, and this has led to a change in management priorities, with hearing conservation increasingly being the goal of therapy.

## Retrosigmoid Approach

The standard practice of one of the authors is to use the retrosigmoid approach to remove small and medium-sized tumors, up to 2 cm in size, in the cerebellopontine angle. Using a rigid endoscope (4 mm or 2.7 mm in diameter) during surgery for small or medium-sized tumors, the surgeon can obtain more accurate information about the relationships between the tumor process and the adjacent structures. Endoscopes are needed to map the anatomical landscape, a great deal of which is normally beyond the rather limited view provided by the microscope.

At the beginning of the surgical procedure, the endoscope allows visualization of: the cerebellar arteries; the medial pole of the tumor and the acousticofacial nerve bundle as it exits the pontomedullary junction; the facial nerve, situated anteriorly, hidden from view and protected by the acoustic nerve; and the trigeminal nerve in the background of the operating field.

## First Case (Figs. 159–162)

The gadolinium-enhanced MRI in this 34-year-old man demonstrated an acoustic tumor of stage II, with a 1-cm extension into the right cerebellopontine angle.

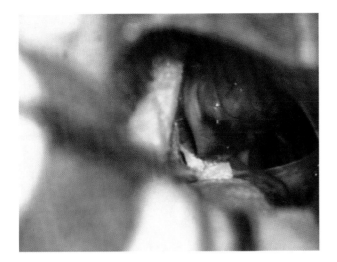

Fig. **159** Operative view using the microscope through a minimally invasive retrosigmoid approach.

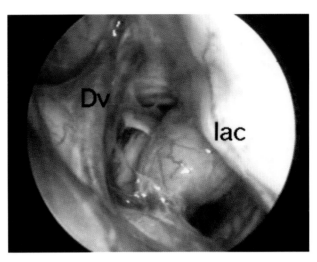

Fig. **160** The acoustic neuroma is inspected with a 4-mm diameter endoscope, which expands the view inside the cerebellopontine angle without contact with the cerebellum or the brain stem.

Dv  Dandy vein
Iac  Internal auditory canal

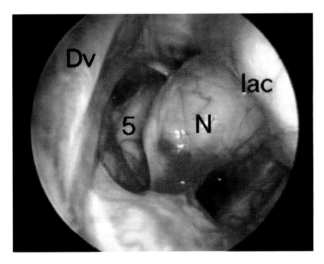

Fig. **161** The following structures are clearly identified: the course of the anterior inferior cerebellar artery and the trigeminal nerve up to the tumor (N).

5    Trigeminal nerve
Dv   Dandy vein
Iac  Internal auditory canal

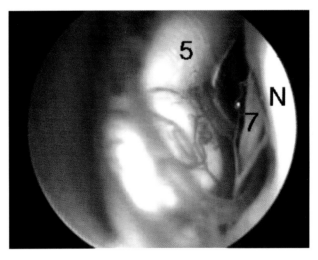

Fig. **162** The tip of the endoscope is positioned above the acoustic neuroma. Exposure of the exact location of the medial end of the facial nerve anterior to the tumor (N), and of the artery between facial and acoustic nerves.

5    Trigeminal nerve
7    Facial nerve

## Second Case (Figs. 163–166)

The gadolinium-enhanced MRI in this 27-year-old woman demonstrated a right stage II acoustic neuroma.

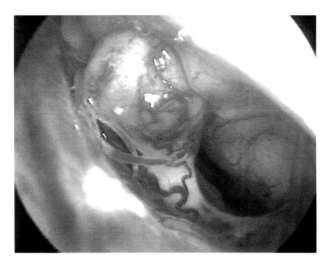

Fig. **163**   Panoramic view of the stage II acoustic neuroma.

Hearing preservation surgery requires bone removal from the posterior lip of the internal auditory canal to be as conservative as possible, to prevent the labyrinth from being entered. Using the retrosigmoid approach, the entrance of the tumor into the porus acusticus provides unquestionable identification of the internal auditory canal. Using a cutting and then a diamond burr, the posterior wall of the internal auditory canal is easily drilled away.

The problem facing the surgeon is to obtain maximum exposure of the intrameatal tumor while at the same time minimizing the risk of inadvertent injury to the labyrinth. From an anatomical viewpoint, the most lateral part of the internal auditory canal exposes the labyrinthine structures, and the surgeon should therefore respect the most lateral 2 mm of the internal auditory canal. Unfortunately, there is no anatomical landmark that could be observed to help avoid injury to the labyrinth. Neither the foramen singulare, the vestibular aqueduct, nor the transverse crest are useful during the surgical procedure.

The most reliable method of reaching the most lateral extent of the internal auditory canal without jeopardizing the inner ear is by using measurements from the patient's CT scan, between the posterior wall of the petrous bone and the labyrinthine structures. The extent of the drilling can then be adjusted according to the radiological data, and can be measured using a burr of known size, or with a graduated instrument.

Usually, the tumor can be rolled out en bloc from the lateral extremity of the internal auditory canal. When the tumor fills the fundus, we use an angled instrument, and the lateral part of the tumor is dissected from medial to lateral and from anterior to posterior, so as to protect the facial and cochlear nerves.

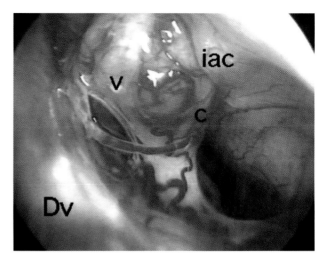

Fig. **164**   Closer view, showing the medial end of the acoustic neuroma. The cochlear nerve is inferior, and the vestibular nerve is superior.

| | | | |
|---|---|---|---|
| c | Cochlear nerve | Iac | Internal auditory canal |
| Dv | Dandy vein | v | Vestibular nerve |

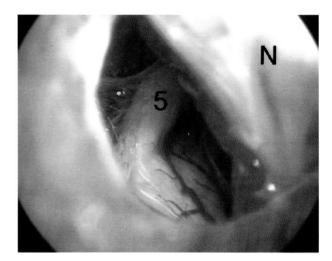

Fig. **165**   Endoscopic view of the trigeminal area.

5  Trigeminal nerve          N  Tumor

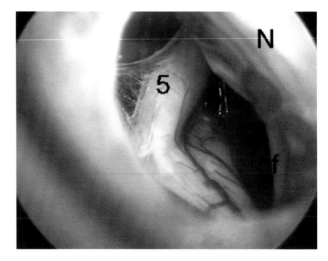

Fig. **166**   Further ahead, the facial nerve (f) is clearly identified anterior to the tumor.

5  Trigeminal nerve          N  Tumor
f  Facial nerve

## Third Case

The gadolinium-enhanced MRI in a 44-year-old man demonstrated an intracanalicular tumor. (Figs. **167–175**)

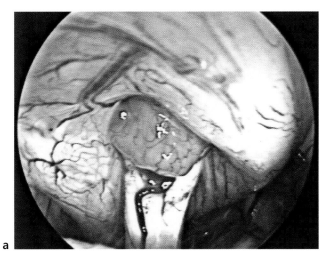

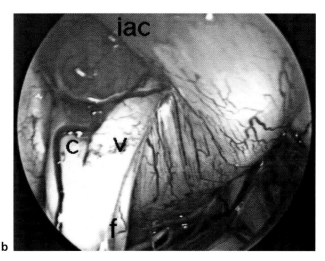

Fig. **167a, b**  Endoscopic views of the acousticofacial nerve bundle in the cerebellopontine angle and the medial part of the intracanalicular tumor at the porus acusticus, allowing an accurate view of the various neural components.

c   Cochlear nerve
f   Facial nerve
iac Internal auditory canal
v   Vestibular nerve

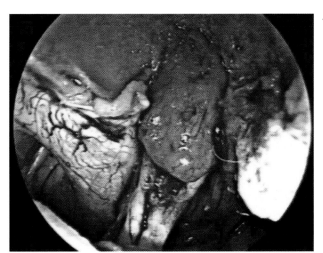

◄ Fig. **168**  Drilling of the posterior wall of the internal auditory canal exposes the entire intracanalicular extent of the tumor. The endoscope allows preservation of the labyrinthine structures.

Fig. **169a, b**  The fundus of the internal auditory canal, which is not visible with an operating microscope, is seen with the endoscope. Both the completeness of the tumor excision and the continuity of the facial (f) and cochlear nerves are checked. There is a small fragment left (N).

c   Cochlear nerve
f   Facial nerve
N   tumor
v   Vestibular nerve

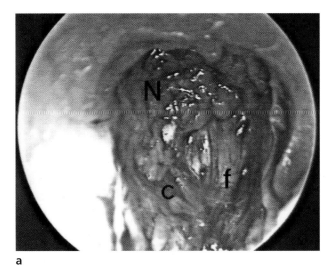

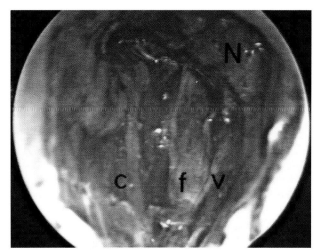

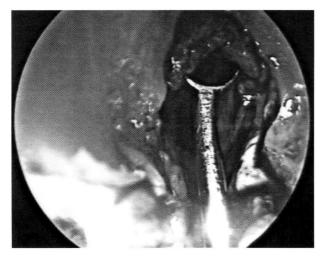

Fig. **170**   Lateral dissection in the internal auditory canal is carried out endoscopically, using curved instruments.

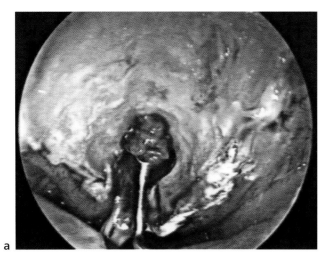

a

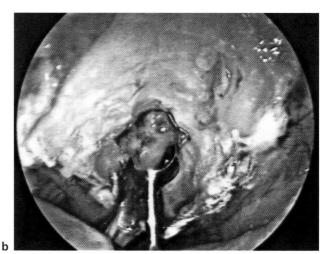

b

Fig. **171a, b**   Using an angled raspatory, the tumor fragment is carefully rolled out of the internal auditory canal.

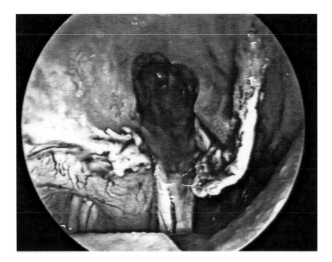

Fig. **172**   The most lateral portion of the internal auditory canal appears to be free of tumor.

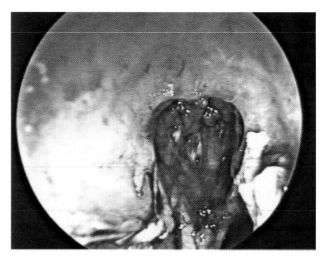

Fig. **173**   However, on a closer endoscopic view, a tiny piece of tumor is seen to remain.

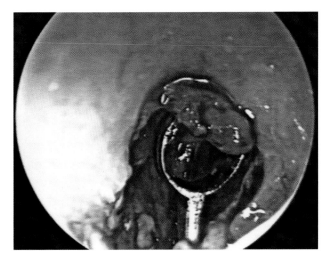

Fig. **174**   The 2-mm tumor (the size of the circular raspatory is 2 mm) is outside the internal auditory canal.

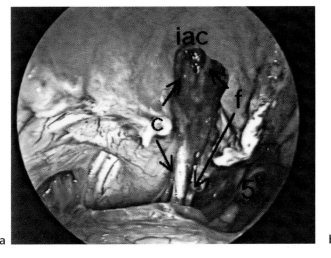

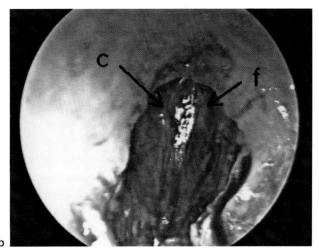

a                                        b

Fig. **175a, b**   Final inspection of the internal auditory canal, which is free of all tumor. The facial and cochlear nerves lie on the anterior wall of the internal auditory canal, and are intimately linked. These relationships must not be disturbed.

5    Trigeminal nerve
c    Cochlear nerve
f    Facial nerve
iac  Internal auditory canal

The principles illustrated here (Figs. **167–175**) can be applied to all small or medium-sized acoustic neuromas, whatever the patient's preoperative hearing threshold. The advantages of the retrosigmoid approach are that less time is required for the surgical approach; there is direct access to the tumor and adjacent structures; there is a possibility of preserving hearing function in 46% of cases. On the other hand, the facial nerve is preserved in 96% (grade I/II, House–Brackmann classification).

The assistance provided by endoscopy in the right retrosigmoid approach is illustrated in Figures **176–179**.

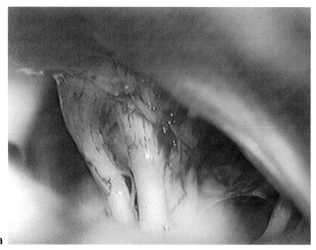
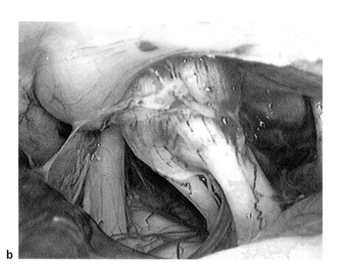

Fig. **176a, b**   A small acoustic neuroma. **a** Operating microscope; **b** Endosopic view.

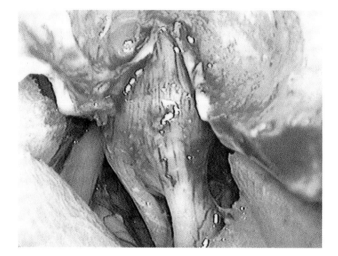

Fig. **177**   A closer view toward the facial nerve and the trigeminal area.

5  Trigeminal nerve
c  Cochlear nerve

f  Facial nerve
v  Vestibular nerve

Fig. **178**   Overview of the tumor after drilling of the internal auditory canal.

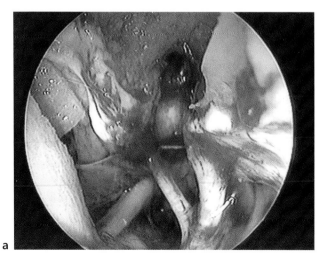
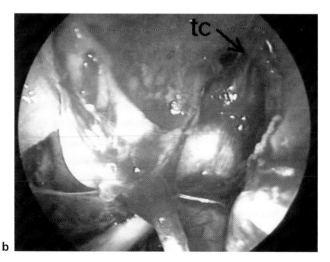

Fig. **179a, b**   Endoscopic inspection of the tumor removal inside the internal auditory canal.

tc  Transverse crest

## Acoustic Neuroma and Hearing Preservation (First Example) (Figs. 180, 181)

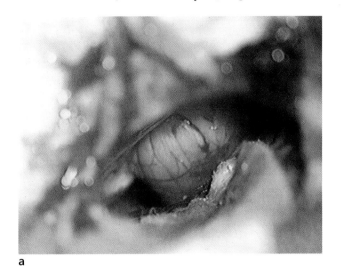

a

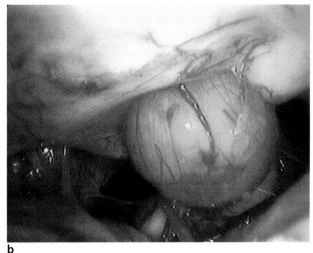

b

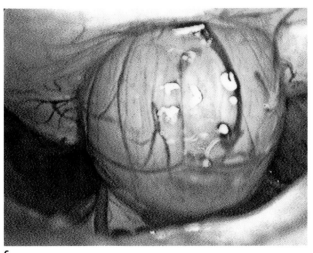

c

Fig. **180** View of a 1.5 cm acoustic neuroma via a left retrosigmoid approach. (**a**) View through the surgical microscope; (**b**) endoscopic view; (**c**) endoscopic view with Digivideo.

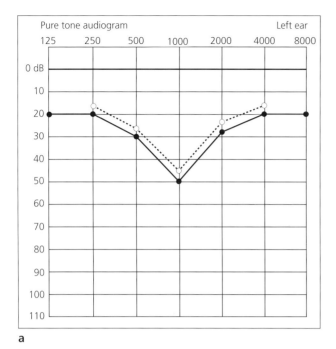

a

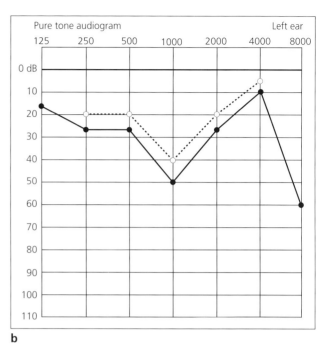

b

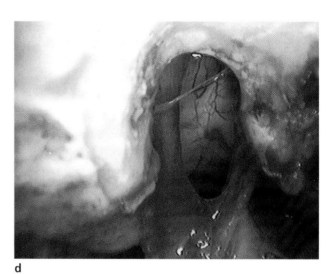

c

d

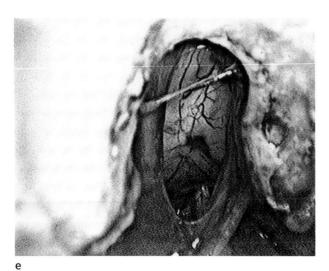

e

Fig. **181a–e**  Preoperative hearing (**a**). Postoperative hearing (**b**). Confirmation of total tumor removal in the internal auditory canal. (**c**) The bottom of the internal auditory canal is not seen through the operative microscope. (**d,e**) With the endoscope, the facial and cochlear nerves are visualized until they penetrate inside the petrous bone.

## Second Example (Fig. 182)

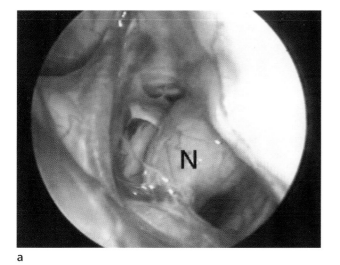

a

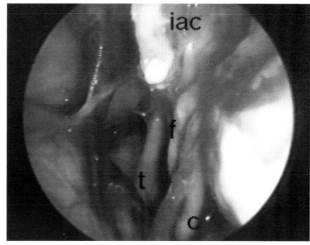

b

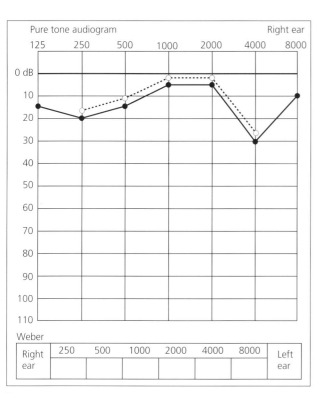

c

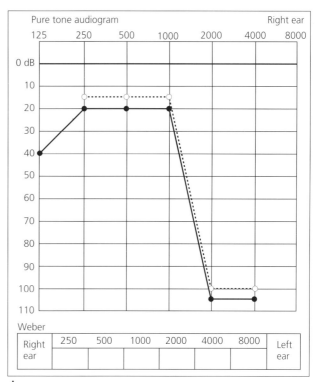

d

Fig. **182a–d**   Preoperative hearing (**c**); postoperative hearing (**d**).

c   Cochlear nerve
f   Facial nerve
iac Internal auditory canal
N   Tumor
t   Trigeminal nerve

**Third Example** (Fig. **183**)

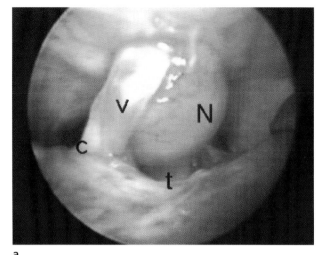

a

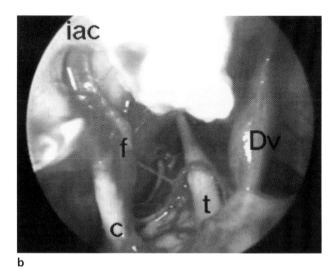

b

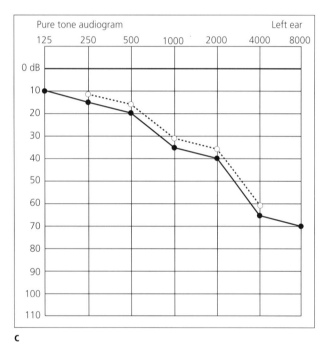

c

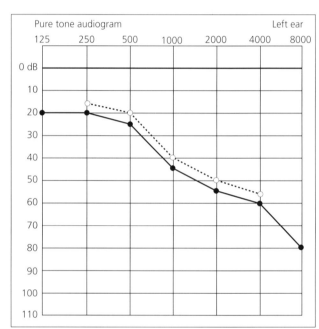

d

Fig. **183a–d**   Preoperative hearing (**c**); postoperative hearing (**d**).

c   Cochlear nerve
Dv   Dandy vein
f   Facial nerve
iac   Internal auditory canal
N   Tumor
t   Trigeminal nerve
v   Vestibular nerve

**Fourth Example** (Fig. **184**)

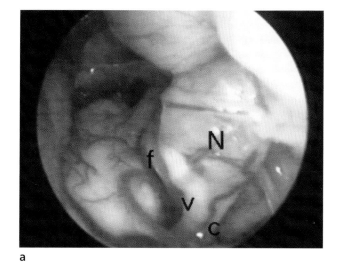

a

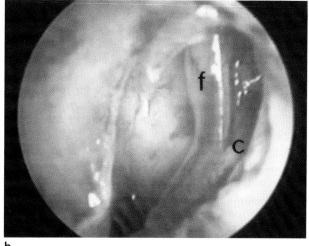

b

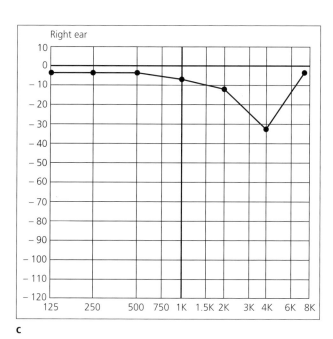

c

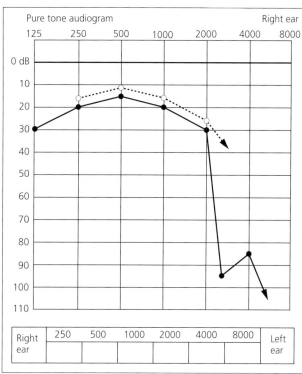

d

Fig. **184a–d**   Preoperative hearing (**c**); postoperative hearing (**d**).

c   Cochlear nerve
f   Facial nerve
N   Tumor
v   Vestibular nerve

## Middle Fossa Approach

The earliest middle fossa approaches were used for exposure of the trigeminal nerve in the treatment of trigeminal neuralgia. The middle fossa procedure has met with widespread use for exposure of the internal auditory canal in the management of facial nerve lesions, selective vestibular neurotomy, and for the removal of tumors.

To expose the internal auditory canal, the temporal craniotomy (approximately 4 × 4 cm) is centered over the ear canal, followed by extradural retraction of the temporal lobe. A specialized retractor is very helpful in maintaining stable temporal lobe elevation. The technique for identifying the plane of the internal auditory canal has been described by House (1964, 1968),

Fisch (1970), and Garcia-Ibanez (1973). Whatever the landmarks used, the superior wall of the internal auditory canal is opened at the deepest point of the exposure towards the porus acusticus, medial to the otic capsule. The lateral portion of the canal is then unroofed.

The middle fossa approach is reserved for intracanalicular acoustic neuromas, or tumors with limited extension (less than 1 cm) into the cerebellopontine angle. The endoscope is used in the same way and for the same purposes in the middle fossa approach as in the retrosigmoid approach.

### Intracanalicular Tumor (First Example)
(Figs. **185–189**)

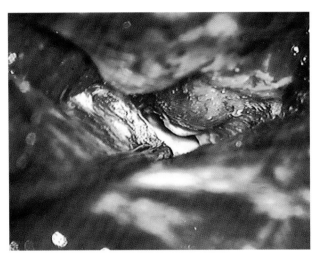

Fig. **185**   Surgical exposure of the acoustic neuroma using a left middle fossa approach.

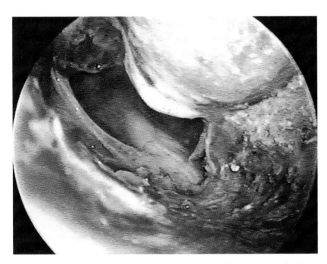

Fig. **186**   The endoscope passes over the tumor before reaching the cerebellopontine angle.

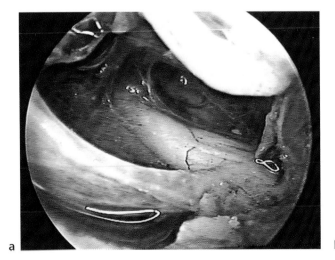

a

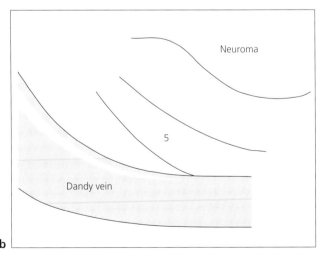

b

Fig. **187a, b**   The Dandy vein and the root of the trigeminal nerve are identified first, and then the medial pole of the acoustic neuroma and the course of the facial nerve.

5   Trigeminal nerve

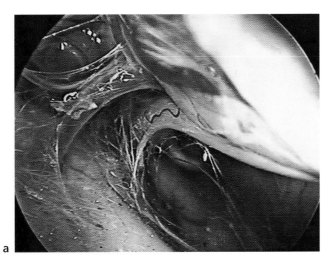

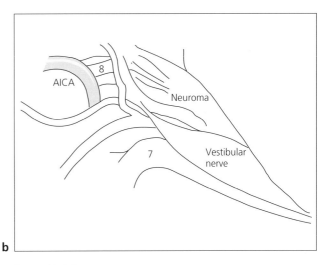

a

b

Fig. **188a, b**  After surgical removal of the acoustic neuroma, the endoscope is used first to inspect the fundus of the internal auditory canal and to confirm the integrity of the facial nerve.

7     Facial nerve
8     Vestibulocochlear nerve
AICA  Anterior inferior cerebellar artery

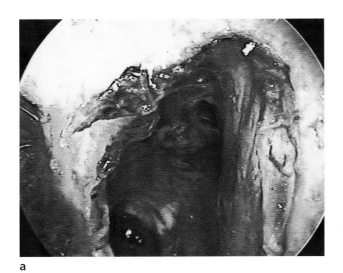

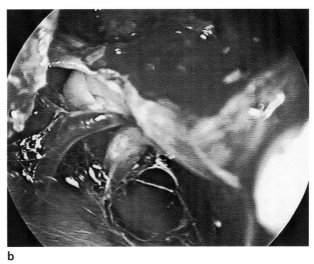

a

b

Fig. **189a–c**  In the cerebellopontine angle, the cochlear and facial nerves are inspected, and between them the anterior inferior cerebellar artery is seen.

7     Facial nerve
8     Vestibulocochlear nerve
AICA  Anterior inferior cerebellar artery

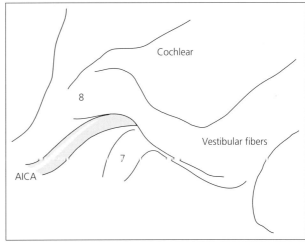

c

## Intracanalicular Tumor (Second Example)
(Figs. **190–194**)

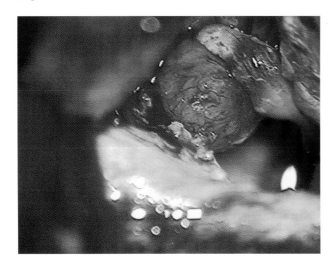

Fig. **190**   Left middle fossa approach. Surgical opening of the internal auditory canal and exposure of the acoustic neuroma.

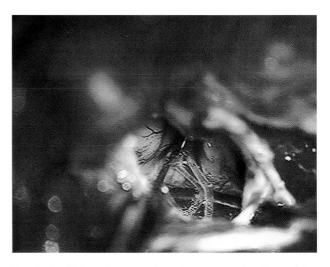

Fig. **191**   Using the operating microscope, the view of the cerebellopontine angle is limited.

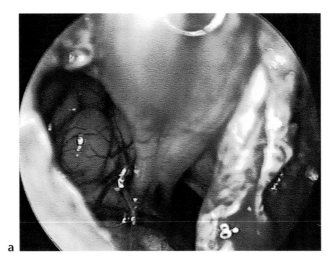

a

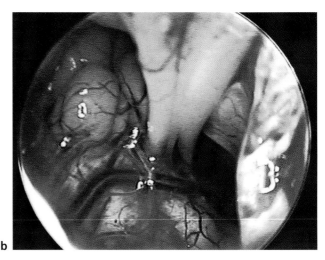

b

Fig. **192a, b**   The same view using a 0° endoscope, diameter 4 mm. The medial part of the acousticofacial nerve bundle and the adjacent vascular structures are clearly identified before the tumor is removed.

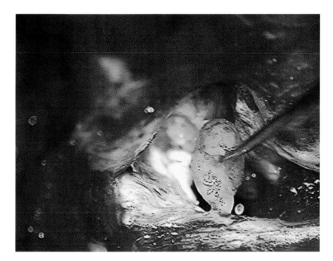

Fig. **193** Surgical view of en-bloc acoustic neuroma removal.

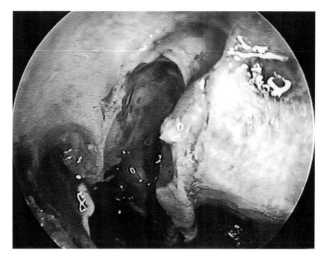

Fig. **194** Endoscopic inspection of the internal auditory canal for any residual tumor. The transverse crest divides the fundus of the internal auditory canal. The facial nerve is hidden and protected by the dura mater of the anterior margin of the internal auditory canal.

## Retrolabyrinthine Approach

The retrolabyrinthine approach was first described by Hitselberger and Pulec (1972), as an approach to the root entry zone of the trigeminal nerve in tic douloureux. It later became a frequently used method of performing vestibular neurotomy (Silverstein 1980) and microvascular decompression (Wiet 1989).

The retrolabyrinthine approach consists of a small posterior fossa craniotomy, between the sigmoid sinus and the otic capsule. It provides limited exposure of

the posterior fossa, confined to the region of the entry zone of the trigeminal nerve and acousticofacial nerve bundle. More lateral structures, such as the porus acusticus and the internal auditory canal, cannot be visualized directly, since they are blocked by the otic capsule. In order to reach and inspect the internal auditory canal, it is necessary first to enlarge the approach posteriorly, removing the bone overlying the sigmoid sinus and 1–2 cm of the retrosigmoid occipital bone; and secondly, to use the endoscopic procedure (Figs. **195–199**).

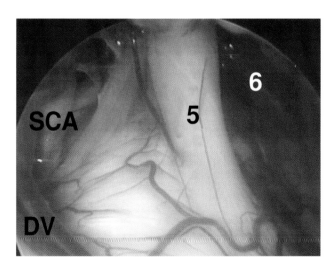

Fig. **195** Endoscopic view of the root entry zone of the trigeminal nerve through a right retrolabyrinthine approach. Note the distance between the superior cerebellar artery and the fifth nerve.

5    Trigeminal nerve
6    Abducent nerve
DV   Dandy vein
SCA  Superior cerebellar artery

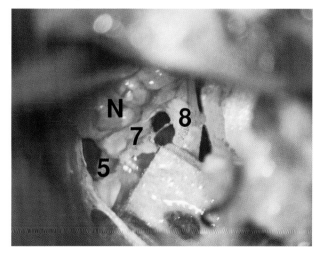

Fig. **196** Surgical view of acoustic neuroma (N) removal using the right retrolabyrinthine approach. The dissection is carried out from medial to lateral. The fifth, seventh, and eighth cranial nerves are identified.

5    Trigeminal nerve
7    Facial nerve
8    Vestibulocochlear nerve

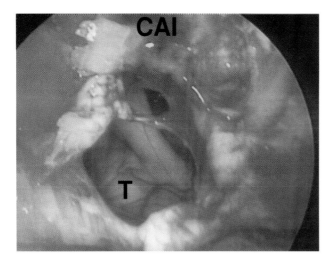

Fig. **197** Endoscopic procedure using a 0° endoscope, diameter 4 mm. After excision of the acoustic neuroma, the brain stem (T), trigeminal nerve, and superior side of the acousticofacial nerve bundle are viewed with the endoscope.

CAI  Internal auditory canal

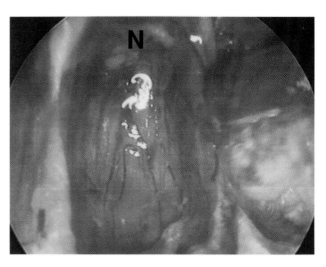

Fig. **198** Endoscopic inspection of the internal auditory canal allows complete exposure of all the intracanalicular components. There is residual tumor (N) filling the lateral recess of the internal auditory canal, which was not visible with the operating microscope.

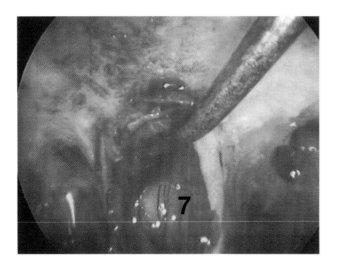

Fig. **199** Assisted endoscopic dissection is carried out using of a 30° angled endoscope and a tip-angled instrument.

7  Facial nerve

## Left Retrolabyrinthine Approach (Figs. 200–202)

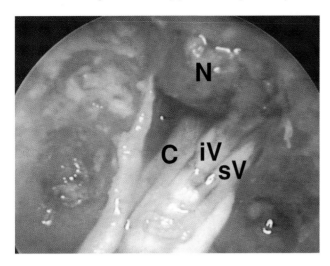

Fig. **200** A small intracanalicular acoustic neuroma (N), arising from the inferior vestibular nerve, is filling the lateral recess of the internal auditory canal.

C Cochlear nerve
iV Inferior vestibular nerve
N Neuroma
sV Superior vestibular nerve

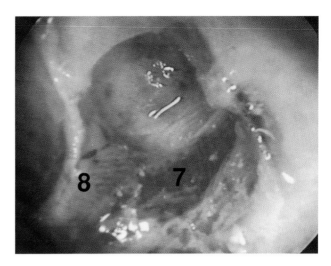

Fig. **201** Partial removal of the acoustic neuroma after sectioning the vestibular nerve. The facial nerve is visualized. The lateral pole of the tumor is adhering to the cochlear nerve, requiring it to be sacrificed in order to achieve complete tumor removal, in spite of the preservation of the labyrinth.

7 Facial nerve
8 Cochlear nerve

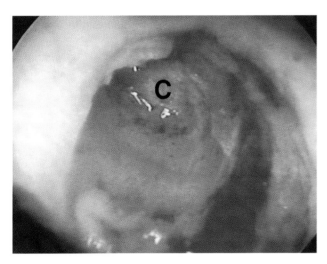

Fig. **202** Endoscopic inspection after assisted endoscopic dissection. The fundus of the internal auditory canal is free of tumor. The facial nerve has been spared from any injury. The cochlear nerve is sectioned, and the cochlear fossa (C) can be visualized.

## Translabyrinthine Approach

The translabyrinthine approach was promoted by House (1964), and was originally used for acoustic neuroma surgery. The endoscopic procedure can be used during two parts of this approach: first, at the beginning of the surgical procedure, using a 0° or a 30° angled endoscope 4 mm in diameter to visualize the relationships between the neural and vascular structures adjacent to the tumor; and secondly, at the end of the surgical procedure, to maximize the exposure of the cerebellopontine angle in order to inspect neural structures and hemostasis.

**Before Tumor Removal** (Figs. **203–206**)

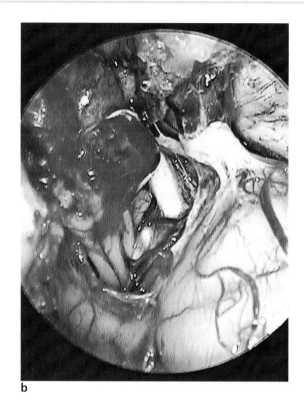

b

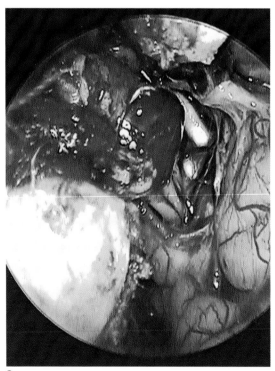

a

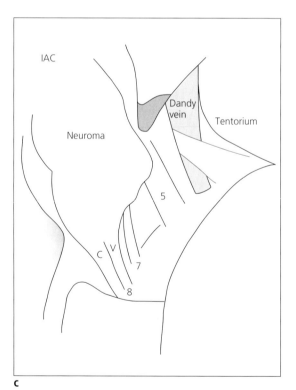

c

Fig. **203a–c** After maximum translabyrinthine bone removal, the opening into the CPA is limited superiorly, to the petrosal sinus, inferiorly, to the jugular bulb; and posteriorly, to the sigmoid sinus. This provides exposure of the whole CPA, including the acoustic neuroma, the lateral aspect of the pons, the ventral surface of the lateral cerebellar hemisphere, the proximal portion of the acousticofacial nerve bundle, and the trigeminal nerve.

5    Trigeminal nerve
7    Facial nerve
8    Vestibulocochlear nerve
IAC  Internal auditory canal
V    Vestibular component of eighth cranial nerve
c    Cochlear component

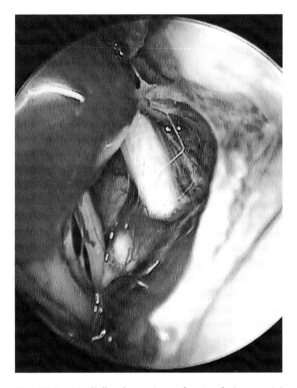

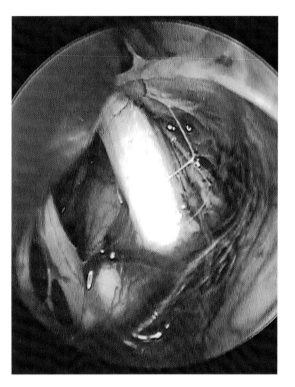

Fig. **204**  Medially, the points of exit of the cranial nerves from the brain stem are clearly visualized. The trigeminal nerve is seen anterior and superior to the tumor. The facial nerve lies medial and anterior to the tumor.

Fig. **205**  Closer view of the brainstem and the root exit zones of the trigeminal and facial nerves. The abducent nerve is visualized in the background.

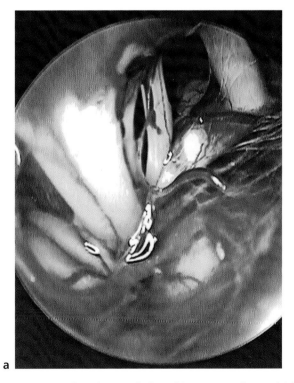

a

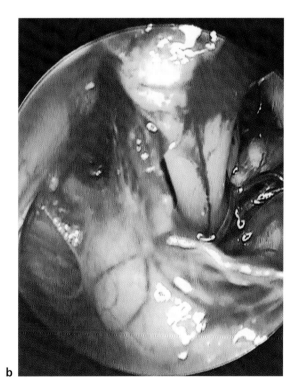

b

Fig. **206a, b**  The vestibulocochlear nerve, from which the tumor arises, is seen medial to the tumor. Anterior and adjacent to the vestibulocochlear nerve runs the nerve of Wrisberg. The flocculus is inferior to the tumor, and there is a loop of the anterior inferior cerebellar artery. The lower cranial nerves are seen in the background, surrounded by the arachnoid sheet. The endoscope provides the surgeon with a map of all the neurovascular components of the CPA, minimizing the need for retraction and dissection.

## After Tumor Removal (Fig. 207)

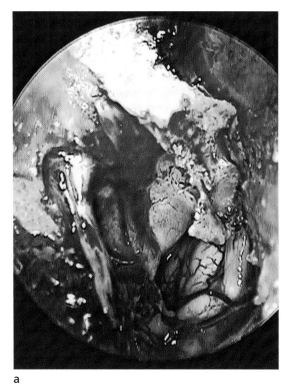

a

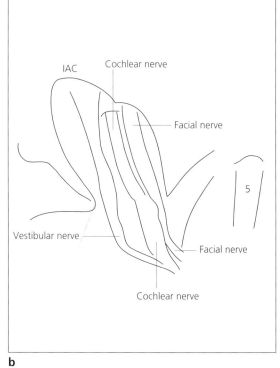

b

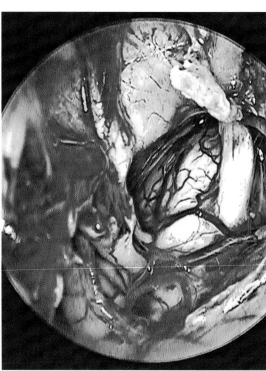

c

d

Fig. **207a–e**   After microdissection of the tumor away from the brain and cranial nerves, an endoscopic inspection is made to check the completeness of tumor removal from the internal auditory canal and cerebellopontine angle. The courses of the cochlear and facial nerves are gradually followed, and the integrity of the nerves is checked. In addition, control of all bleeding vessels is ensured.

5    Trigeminal nerve
IAC  Internal auditory canal

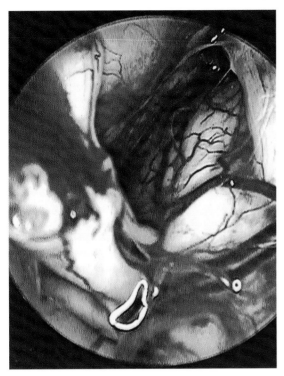

207e

## Right Translabyrinthine Approach: Small Tumors (Figs. 208–212)

Using a 0° endoscope with a diameter of 4 mm, the relationships between the acoustic neuroma and the adjacent structures can be evaluated.

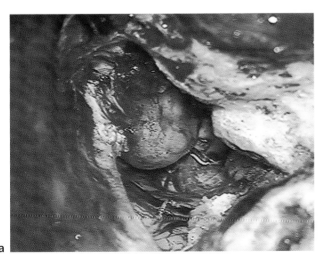
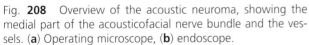

a

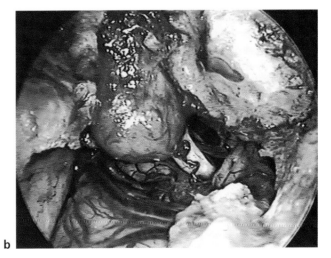

b

Fig. **208**  Overview of the acoustic neuroma, showing the medial part of the acousticofacial nerve bundle and the vessels. (**a**) Operating microscope, (**b**) endoscope.

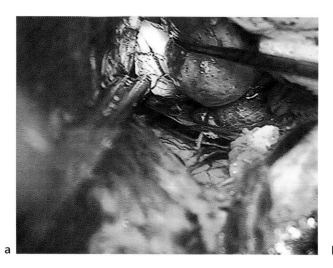

Fig. **209**   The trigeminal nerve anterior and superior to the tumor. (**a**) Operating microscope, (**b**) endoscope.

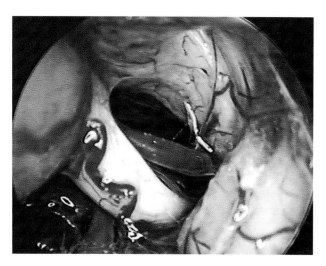

Fig. **210**   With a 30° angled endoscope close to the medial pole of the tumor, the view is directed posteriorly; flocculus and lower cranial nerves are under vision.

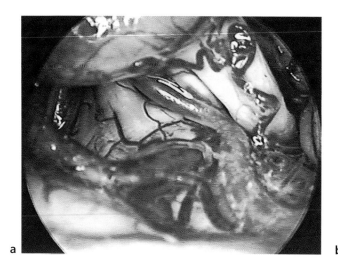

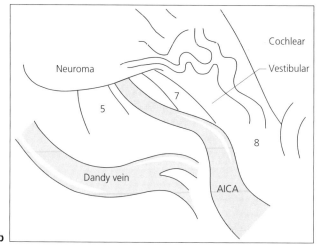

Fig. **211a, b**   The eighth nerve, with the cochlear and vestibular components; the facial nerve anteriorly and the anterior inferior cerebellar artery are definitively identified.

5      Trigeminal nerve
7      Facial nerve
8      Vestibulocochlear nerve
AICA   Anterior inferior cerebellar artery

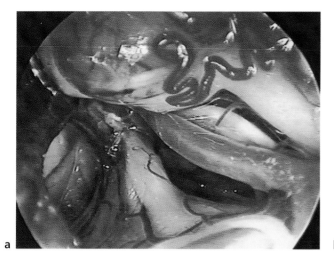

a

b

Fig. **212a, b**   With a 30° angled endoscope, the view is directed anteriorly; trigeminal area, site of the facial nerve and course of the anterior inferior cerebellar artery are under vision.

5     Trigeminal nerve
7     Facial nerve
8     Vestibulocochlear nerve
AICA   Anterior inferior cerebellar artery

## Right Translabyrinthine Approach: Medium-Sized Tumors (First Example) (Figs. **213–218**)

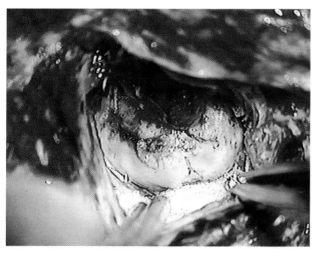

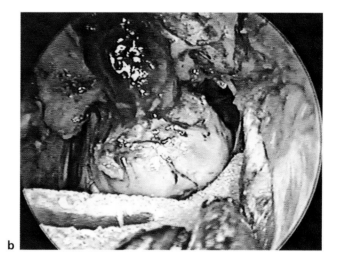

a

b

Fig. **213a, b**   (**a**) Operating microscope; (**b**) endoscope.

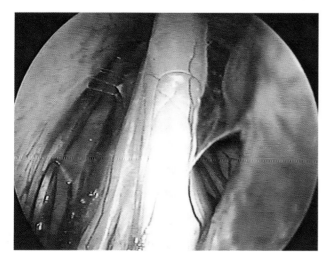

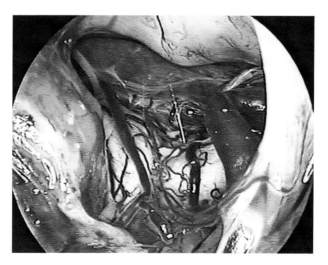

Fig. **214**   Above the tumor, there is no distortion of the trigeminal nerve; the superior cerebellar artery, the trochlear nerve, and the tentorium are seen.

Fig. **215**   Below the tumor, the posterior inferior cerebellar artery and glossopharyngeal nerve are seen; anteriorly lie the abducent nerve and the anterior inferior cerebellar artery.

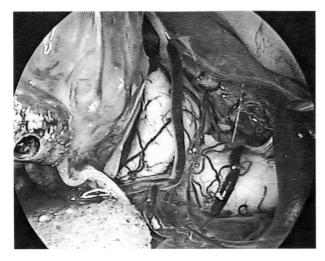

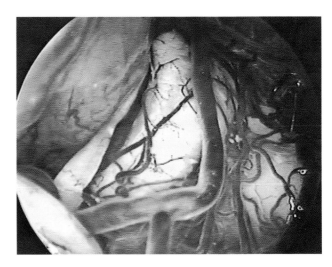

Fig. **216**   At the inferior part of the acoustic neuroma, the root exit zone of the facial nerve is stretched by the tumor; in the background lies the basilar artery.

Fig. **217**   A closer view of the facial nerve. A vascular loop from the anterior inferior cerebellar artery is in contact with the medial part of the tumor.

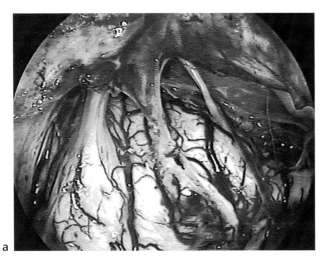

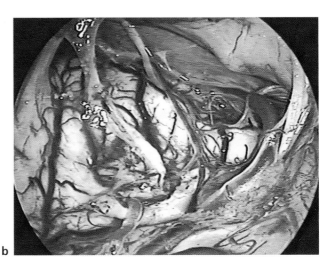

Fig. **218a, b**   Endoscopic inspection after tumor removal. The facial nerve is intact from the brain stem to the fundus of the internal auditory canal. There is no residual tumor or bleeding within the cerebellopontine angle.

## Left Translabyrinthine Approach: Medium-Sized Tumor (Second Example) (Figs. 219–222)

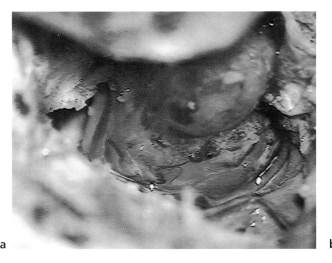

a

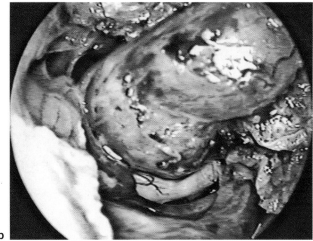

b

Fig. **219** The acoustic tumor is distorting the trigeminal nerve. (**a**) Operating microscope; (**b**) endoscopic view.

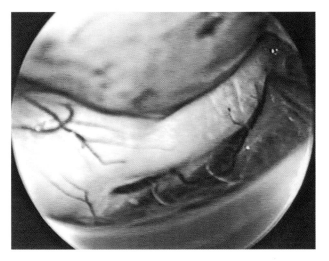

Fig. **220** Above the acoustic neuroma, there is distortion of the trigeminal nerve around the tumor.

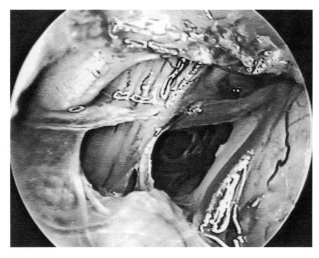

Fig. **221** Below the acoustic neuroma, the anterior inferior cerebellar artery is attached to the eighth nerve and the lower cranial nerves.

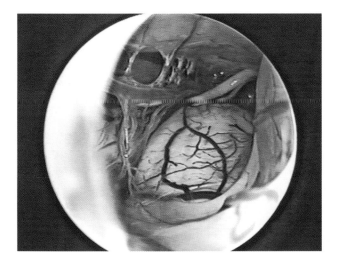

Fig. **222** A closer view. The tip of the endoscope is between the acoustic neuroma and the lower cranial nerves. The root entry zone of the eighth nerve and the root exit zone of the seventh nerve are clearly identified.

## Left Translabyrinthine Approach: Medium-Sized Tumor (Third Example) (Figs. 223–225)

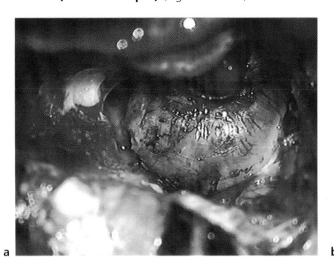

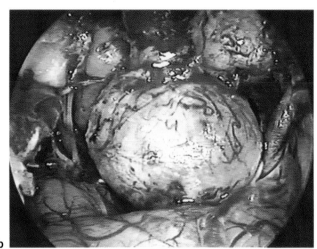

Fig. **223a, b**    (**a**) Operating microscope; (**b**) endoscope.

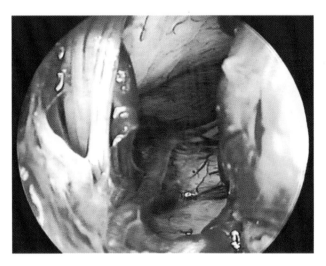

Fig. **224**    Below the acoustic neuroma and above the lower cranial nerves, the root exit zone of the facial nerve is circled by a loop of the anterior inferior cerebellar artery.

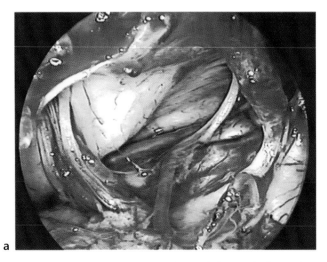

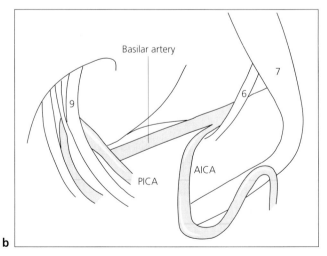

Fig. **225a, b**    Endoscopic checking of the cerebellopontine angle after tumor removal.

6      Abducent nerve
7      Facial nerve
9      Glossopharyngeal nerve
AICA   Anterior inferior cerebellar artery
PICA   Posterior inferior cerebellar artery

## Right Translabyrinthine Approach: Large Tumors (Neurofibromatosis) (Figs. 226–227)

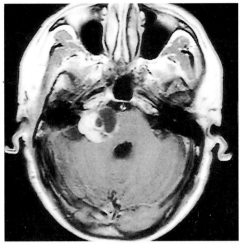

a

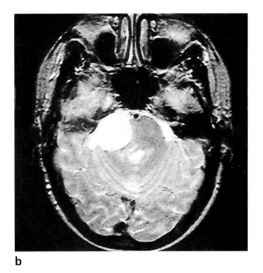

b

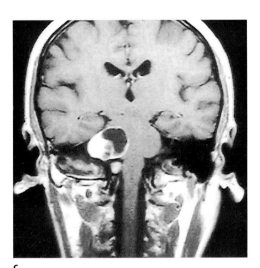

c

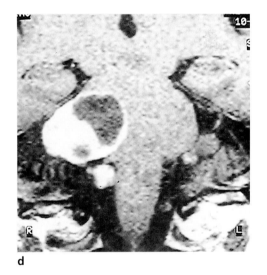

d

Fig. **226a–d**   Imaging assessment. Right CPA cystic acoustic schwannoma. (**a, c, d**) Post gadolinium T1 images in the axial and coronal planes; (**b**) axial T2 image; and (**c, d**) homogeneously enhanced schwannoma arising from the lower cranial nerves.

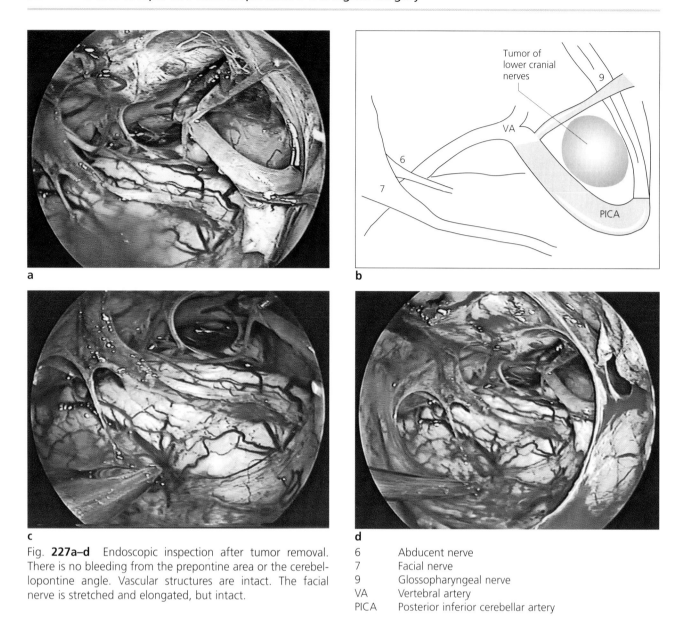

a

b

c

d

Fig. **227a–d** Endoscopic inspection after tumor removal. There is no bleeding from the prepontine area or the cerebellopontine angle. Vascular structures are intact. The facial nerve is stretched and elongated, but intact.

6      Abducent nerve
7      Facial nerve
9      Glossopharyngeal nerve
VA     Vertebral artery
PICA   Posterior inferior cerebellar artery

# References

Arriaga M, Chen D, Fukushima T. Individualizing hearing preservation in acoustic neuroma surgery. Laryngoscope 1997; 107: 1043–7.

Charachon R, Lavielle JP, Chirossel JP. Neurinomes de l'acoustique. Encyclopedie Medico-Chirurgicale (EMC) (Paris: Elsevier) Oto-Rhino-Laryngologie 1997; 20–250–A10: 180.

Colleaux B, Chays A, Dubreuil C, Magnan J, Boudud B. Neurinome de l'acoustique et conservation de l'audition. J Fr Otorhinolaryngol 1994; 43: 101–5.

Darrouzet V, Guerin J, Aouad N, Dutkiewicz J, Blayney N, Bebear JP. The widened retrolabyrinthine approach: a new concept in acoustic neuroma surgery. J Neurosurg 1997; 86: 818–21.

Darrouzet V, Guerin J, Portmann D, et al. La voie retro-labyrinthique élargie. Application à la chirurgie du neurinome de l'acoustique. Rev Laryngol 1993; 114: 207–11.

Fisch U. Transtemporal surgery of the internal auditory canal. Adv Otorhinolaryngol 1970; 17: 203.

Garcia-Ibaneze. Cirurgia del conducto auditivo interno. Acta Otorhinolaryngol Esp (Madrid) 1973; 8: 219-223.

Gardner G, Robertson J, Clark W. Acoustic tumor management. Am J Otol 1983; 5: 87–108.

Haid C, Wigand M. Advantages of the enlarged middle cranial fossa approach in acoustic neuroma surgery: a review. Acta Otolaryngol 1992; 112: 387–407.

Hecht C, Honrubia V, Wiet R, Sims S. Hearing preservation after acoustic neuroma resection with tumor size used as a clinical prognosticator. Laryngoscope 1997; 107: 1122–6.

Hitselberger WE, Pulec JL. Trigeminal nerve retrolabyrinthine selective section. Arch Otolaryngol 1972; 96: 412-415.

House WF. Historical review and problem of acoustic neuroma. Arch Otolaryngol 1964; 80: 617-756.

House WF. Acoustic neuroma: case summaries. Arch Otolaryngol 1968; 88: 586–91.

McKennan K. Endoscopy of the internal auditory canal during hearing conservation acoustic tumor surgery. Am J Otol 1993; 14: 259–62.

Magnan J, Chays A, Bremond G. Hearing preservation by the retrosigmoid approach. In: Tos M, Thomsen J, eds. Acoustic neuroma. Amsterdam: Kugler, 1992: 641–5.

Martin C, Prades JM, Loubeyre A, Detsouli M. La voie retro-labyrinthique élargie. Intérît dans la chirurgie du neurinome de l'acoustique avec tentative de conservation auditive. Rev Laryngol 1995; 116: 119–22.

Mazzoni A, Calabrese V, Moschini L. Residual and recurrent acoustic neuroma in hearing preservation procedures: neuro-radiologic and surgical findings. Skull Base Surg 1996; 6: 105–12.

Sanna M, Saleh E, Panizza B. Color atlas of acoustic neurinoma microsurgery. Stuttgart: Thieme, 1997.

Silverstein, Norrel H. Retrolabyrinthine surgery: A direct approach to the cerebellopontine angle. Otolaryngol Head Neck Surg 1980; 88: 462-469.

Slattery W, Brackmann D, Hitselberger W. Middle fossa approach for hearing preservation with acoustic neuromas. Am J Otol 1997; 18: 596–601.

Sterkers JM, Charachon R, Sterkers O. Acoustic neuroma and skull base surgery. Amsterdam. Kugler, 1996.

Tos M, Thomsen J. Acoustic neuroma. Amsterdam: Kugler, 1992.

Wiet R, Schramm D, Kazan R. The retrolabyrinthine approach and vascular loop. Laryngoscope 1989; 99: 1035-1039.

## ■ Lower Cranial Nerve Neuroma
(Figs. **228–230**)

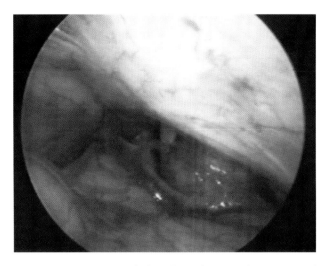

Fig. **228**   Neuromas of the glossopharyngeal, vagus, and spinal accessory nerves account for fewer than 1% of cerebellopontine lesions, and may either be isolated or occur with neurofibromatosis. Overview of the CPA with a tumor in the lower cranial nerve area.

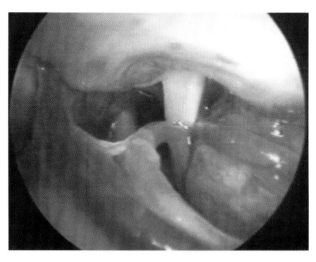

Fig. **229**   Distortion of the acousticofacial nerve bundle by a tumor arising from the lower cranial nerve area.

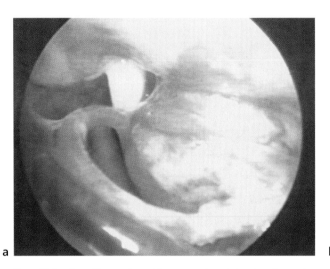

a

Fig. **230a, b**   Closer view. The tumor is originating from the pars nervosa of the jugular foramen.

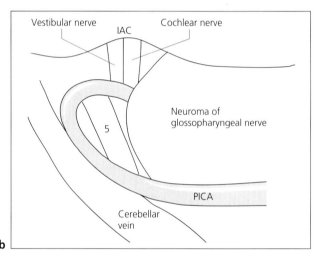

b

5      Trigeminal nerve
IAC    Internal auditory canal
PICA   Posterior inferior cerebellar artery

### Reference

Mazzoni A, Sanna M, Saleh E, Achilli U. Lower cranial nerve schwannomas involving the jugular foramen. Ann Otol Rhinol Laryngol 1997; 106: 370–9.

# Cholesteatoma

The incidence of cholesteatoma of the cerebellopontine angle is between 2% and 6% of CPA lesions. Facial pain, facial paresis, and hemifacial spasm are the common presenting symptoms. Unilateral sensorineural hearing loss is a less frequent finding.

### First Case (Retrosigmoid Approach)
(Figs. 231–233)

A 36-year-old woman presented with left hemifacial spasm.

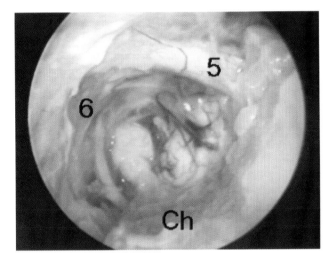

Fig. **231** There is CPA cholesteatoma surrounding the cranial nerves, and adhering to these structures and to the brain stem. Due to the lesion's propensity to penetrate into the substance of the nerve, incomplete surgical removal is common, and there is a high risk of recurrence.

5    Trigeminal nerve
6    Abducent nerve
Ch   Cholesteatoma

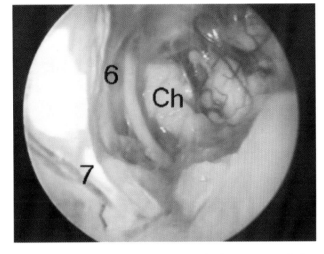

Fig. **232** Using an endoscope provides better appreciation of the extent of the cholesteatoma. The cholesteatoma involves the whole cerebellopontine angle, and has spread to the prepontine area, inducing major distortion of the facial nerve which runs adjacent to the lower cranial nerves.

6    Abducent nerve
7    Facial nerve
Ch   Cholesteatoma

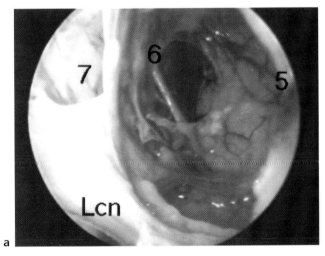

a

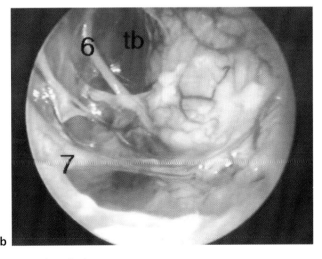

b

Fig. **233a, b**    After meticulous peeling of the thin matrix surrounding the keratin and adhering to the neural structures, the completeness of the surgical excision and preservation of the neurovascular components are confirmed endoscopically.

5    Trigeminal nerve
6    Abducent nerve
7    Facial nerve
Lcn  Lower cranial nerves
tb   Trunk of the basilar artery

## Second Case (Modified Transcochlear Approach, Type A) (Figs. 234–238)

Right cholesteatoma of the petrous apex and cerebellopontine angle.

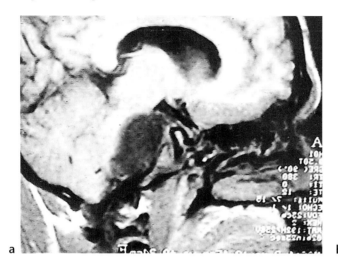
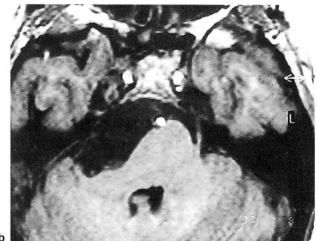

Fig. **234a, b**   Imaging assessment, post gadolinium sagittal (**a**) and axial (**b**). Sections show a low signal tumor with linear high signal lesions scattered through the mass, highly suggestive of right CPA congenital cholesteatoma.

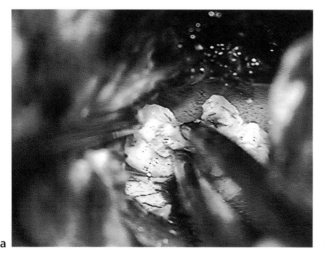
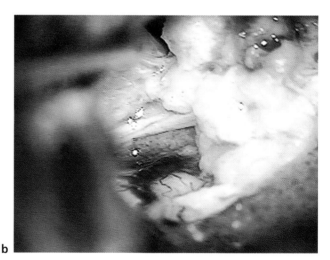

Fig. **235a, b**   Removal of the cholesteatoma

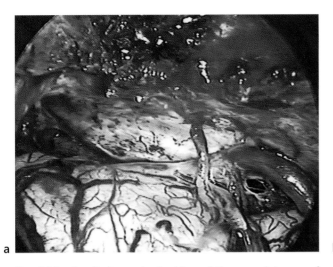

a

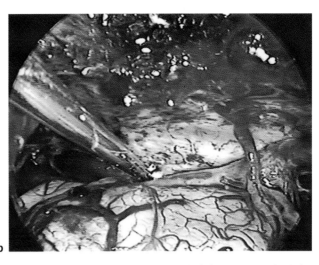

b

Fig. **236a, b** Endoscopic checking of the completeness of the removal. (**a**) Prepontine cistern area. (**b**) Suction–irrigation to clean the basilar artery. The trigeminal nerve lies superiorly, and the vertebrobasilar junction and abducent nerve lie inferiorly.

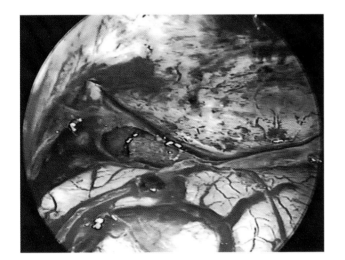

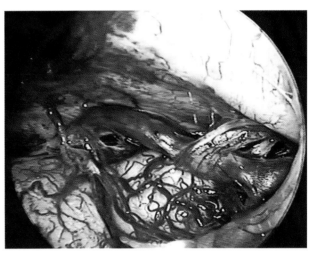

Fig. **237** The deepest view, showing Surgicel around the basilar artery and visualization of the contralateral trigeminal nerve.

Fig. **238** The area of the lower cranial nerves and hypoglossal nerve.

## References

Doyle K, De La Cruz A. Cerebellopontine angle epidermoids: results of surgical treatment. Skull Base Surg 1996, 6: 27–33.

Sanna M, Mazzoni A, Saleh E, Taibah A, Russo A. Lateral approaches to the median skull base through the petrous bone: the system of the modified transcochlear approach. J Laryngol Otol 1994; 108: 1035–43.

# Index